PROVIDER OF
LAST RESORT

PROVIDER OF
LAST RESORT

THE STORY OF THE CLOSURE OF THE
PHILADELPHIA GENERAL HOSPITAL

DONNA GENTILE O'DONNELL

Camino Books, Inc.
Philadelphia

Manufactured in the United States of America

1 2 3 4 5 08 07 06 05

Library of Congress Cataloging-in-Publication Data

O'Donnell, Donna Gentile.
  Provider of last resort : the story of the closure of Philadelphia General Hospital / Donna Gentile O'Donnell.
    p. ; cm.
  Includes bibliographical references.
  ISBN 0-940159-96-1 (alk. paper)
  1. Philadelphia General Hospital--History. 2. Public hospitals—Pennsylvania—Philadelphia—History. 3. Hospital closures—Pennsylvania—Philadelphia—History. 4. Poor—Medical care—Pennsylvania—Philadelphia—History. [DNLM: 1. Philadelphia General Hospital. 2. Health Facility Closure—history—Philadelphia. 3. Health Facility Closure—history—United States. 4. Hospitals, Municipal—history—Philadelphia. 5. Hospitals, Municipal—history—United States. 6. Financing, Government—Philadelphia. 7. Financing, Government--United States. 8. Health Services Accessibility—economics—Philadelphia. 9. Health Services Accessibility--economics—United States. 10. Medical Indigency—Philadelphia. 11. Medical Indigency—United States. WX 28 AP4 O26p 2005] I. Title.

  RA982.P5G363 2005
  362.11'0974811--dc22   2005007400

Cover and interior design: Jerilyn Bockorick

This book is available at a special discount on bulk purchases for promotional, business, and educational use.

Publisher
Camino Books, Inc.
P.O. Box 59026
Philadelphia, PA 19102

www.caminobooks.com

Contents

Acknowledgments

Converting this dissertation into a usable, readable book was a considerable challenge—one that could not have been accomplished without the patience and skill of my editor, Brad Fisher; and my publisher, Edward Jutkowitz, and Barbara Gibbons, of Camino Books. This conversion respects the unique experience of writing a dissertation. Hundreds of hours are spent poring over thousands of pages of archives, notes, documents, books, articles, unpublished dissertations, and interview transcripts, and laboring to condense them into a substantial document presenting a good argument and a cogent point of view. And the process of engaging the work of the dissertation—the research and collaboration—requires extensive involvement with many people who commit their time and talent to the effort.

No one has been more fortunate than I to have Dr. Karen Buhler-Wilkerson chair my dissertation committee and guide my program of research. Karen is a superb historian and an egalitarian educator, with all that that implies. She first raised the PGH closure as an overlooked area of inquiry and research. The idea "landed," and I never looked back. Dr. Julie Fairman, also a member of my committee and another truly remarkable historian, has a fine eye for detail and asked key questions as I pursued a full and fair explanation of the closure. I always looked forward to our "coffee and counsel" sessions. Julie's laser-like focus made me a better researcher. And finally, the amazing Dr. Ted Hershberg, who has long been regarded as a local politics and public policy expert, took great pains to help me keep my eye on the ball, and make sure that this work was both factually accurate and a political story worth telling. My committee has been worth its weight in gold, providing guidance, support, momentum, and encouragement throughout this long, arduous process. I am deeply grateful.

Special thanks to Dr. Claire Fagin, who was an ongoing source of encouragement, and who also co-chaired my almost-successful campaign for City Council in 1999. Claire sets the gold standard for the discipline, single-handedly redefining accomplishment and opportunity by breaking old rules, new ground, and glass ceilings. Thanks also to so many other PENN faculty and staff, present and past, who made contributions, large and small, to my academic life. They include Dr. Anne Keane; Dr. Lorraine Tulman; Dr. Charles Rosenberg; Dr. Drew Faust; Dr. Janet Tighe; Dr. Neville Strumpf; Dr. Susan Gennaro; Dr. Roz Watts; Dr. Joan Lynaugh; Dr. Wanda Mohr; Dr. Linda Aiken; our resident "genius," Dr. Sarah Kagan; the late Dr. Barbara Lowry; Joanne Murray; and Christina Costanzo Clark.

Interviewing key sources knowledgeable about city government, PGH, the closure, or a related area was an important area of inquiry. Sometimes these interviews were brief. Some led to more extensive and illuminating sources and interviews. Many people gave generously of their time to help me sort out the complexities, political and otherwise, that contributed to this monumental event and decision in the life and history of Philadelphia, and the delivery of health care. They include Hillel "Hilly" Levinson, Lt. Anthony Fulwood, Tom Leonard, Martin "Marty" Weinberg, Walt D'Alessio, Jim Baumbach, Ernest Zeger, Barry Savitz, Frank O'Donnell, Stephanie Stachniewicz, Lenora Berson, Dr. Lewis Polk, Health Commissioner John Domzalski, Eileen Kelly, Isador "Izzy" Kranzel, Dr. Walter Lear, Commissioner Joe Rizzo, Duncan Van Dusen, Tina Weintraub, Craig Schelter, Sal Paolantonio, and Councilman Frank Rizzo, Jr. Special thanks also to Betsy Weiss from the Center for the Study of Nursing History; Amey Hutchins from the University of Pennsylvania Library Archives; Rich Fraser from the College of Physicians Library and Archives; Donald Cramp from the Hospitals and Higher Educations Authority; Andrew Wigglesworth from the Delaware Valley Health Care Council; Kathy Carlson-Mebus from the Hospital Association of Pennsylvania; Ward Childs from the City of Philadelphia Archives; and former Health Commissioner Dr. Lewis Polk, for the use of his personal archive, which contained reports and documents that no longer exist in any other archive.

I also want to thank Jeffrey Ray from the Atwater Kent Museum, along with David Rasner and Gardner Cadwalader, who serve on the board of the Atwater Kent, for their critical assistance in placing the portrait of Alice Fisher, the founder of the first training school for nurses at PGH, on renewable loan to the Center for the Study of Nursing History at the University of Pennsylvania. Their willingness to help relocate Alice into a new home was, and is, much appreciated. It was the best serendipitous finding and outcome of my research.

I have the good fortune to have a cadre of friends and colleagues who cheered me on over the six years it took to bring my dissertation studies to a successful conclusion. They include Margaret Swisher; Ellen and Jimmy Lutz; Cherie Patricelli; Barbara Mallory; Barbara Hafer, State Treasurer of the Commonwealth of Pennsylvania; Kelly Preski; Chris Ann Szep; Gloria McNeal; Mark Alan Hughes; Michael Karp; Harvil Eaton; Steve Altschuler (who also helped me sort out the CHOP/PGH geography and time line); my dear friend Justice Sandra Schultz Newman; and my doctoral cohort colleagues, Eileen Alexy, Hilaire Thompson, Meg Bourbonniere, and Pam Jackson-Malik. My colleagues at the *Daily Pennsylvanian*, especially my editors Eliot Sherman and Steve Brauntuch, provided much-needed comic relief in our collective PENN-life...thanks for that.

I am also grateful to my friends and colleagues at the Eastern Technology Council and PA Early Stage Partners, especially Rob McCord and Dianne Strunk...thanks for being in my corner. Rob, who recruited me to the Council with the promise, "I'll nominally be your boss, and you'll tell me what to do," was true to his word, and has been the best mentor and colleague I could have imagined. A most special thanks to my friend and colleague, Pamela "Pammy" Seitzer (better known as "Field Marshall Seitzer"), whose invaluable editing assistance in addressing technical issues in the chapter rewrites was critical to the final product. For that, and for so many other reasons, I am deeply grateful.

I am thankful to my parents, who always encouraged me, and whose pride in my work means so much to me. I am also grateful to my stepson Casey, with whom I have often commiserated as we shared the joys and sufferings of our respective doctoral programs, and who has been a source of ongoing inspiration to me. Both of us are blessed to have life partners—he, my daughter-in-law Sunshine, and I, his father—without whom our doctoral experiences, and lives, would be diminished.

Finally, my thanks to my husband, Bob O'Donnell—the most intellectually able, decent man I know. His insights into applied public policy and public finance helped me crystallize my thinking and frame the implications for PGH. During these six years, he's been my best critic, sounding board, advisor, and supporter. While I whaled away at my keyboard at all hours, he made me dozens of pots of soup and hundreds of cups of tea over the long weeks and months and years of writing and rewriting and revising. His love and affection (along with great soup) have sustained me throughout. I couldn't have done this without you.

Special Thanks

This book is supported in part by the Philadelphia General Hospital Alumni Association, who will celebrate their final gathering in May 2005 as they formally decommission their organization. The Alumni Association has kept the sprit of PGH alive well beyond the closing of the doors of Philadelphia's only public hospital in 1977, and also made much of the research for this book possible. I am deeply grateful for the assistance of so many. Special thanks also to the Philadelphia Hospital and Higher Education Authority, the Eastern Technology Council, and the Drexel University College of Medicine for their support. The royalties from this book will support the Children's Hospital of Philadelphia and the Center for the Study of Nursing History at the University of Pennsylvania.

Introduction

In 1977, when the last patient from Philadelphia General Hospital (PGH) was transferred out through the wrought-iron gates, the end of an era was signaled. Preceding the closure, many forces, large and small, contributed ultimately to the fate of PGH—among them, a political roller-coaster ride that spanned decades; an epic public relations battle; and a major realignment of federal funding streams, which had unintended public policy consequences.

The research for this book made it clear that no one worldview would emerge from the long shadow that Philadelphia General Hospital cast over the life of the city. To some, it was the best hospital in the world. To others, it was the worst. To some, PGH was a remarkable institution that fell on hard times. To others, it was the only place black Philadelphians felt comfortable going to because of its early nondiscrimination policy, which preceded the civil rights legislation of the 1960's. To some, Frank Rizzo was the racist mayor who closed the only hospital that black folks had. To others, Frank Rizzo was the mayor who had the courage to close the worst hospital in the city and force the other hospitals to open their doors wider toward equal treatment.

The institutional and political battles that ensued over the last two decades of Philadelphia General Hospital's existence set the stage for its undoing. What is clear is that PGH did much to shape the development of health care delivery in many important ways, namely, through the synergy between clinical research and the practice of medicine under William Osler; the development of organized nursing in acute care under Alice Fisher; and its embedded notions of social obligation to care for the sick, the needy, and the poor, which found expression in care delivered for those who sought the refuge PGH offered.

In the early 1700's, before the America we know came to be, notions of the "worthy poor" and European-rooted traditions of benevolence served as the underpinnings of pre-American society. It was in this pre–nation state context that the earliest incarnation of the Philadelphia General Hospital, as an almshouse, emerged. Over the centuries that followed, until its closing in 1977, PGH, in all its iterations, stood for "care and cure." But by the time PGH closed, even its strongest supporters and stalwart believers faced insurmountable odds against the survival of this once-noble institution. At the zenith of its institutional life, with 4,000 beds and its own fire department, PGH was a small city unto itself. Resting on 87 acres, PGH became a center of international excellence in science, research, and patient care.

Over time, the health care delivery system expanded and matured, and Philadelphia General Hospital began to lose its luster as a leading-edge entity. Fiscal pressures, bureaucratic complexity, and political expediency; the rearrangement of funding streams and institutional relationships; the forward march of science and research in a changing marketplace; the reorientation of social and institutional structures, including desegregation, the rise of the nonprofit hospital sector, and the creation of the Philadelphia Hospitals Authority, which made tax-exempt financing available for the first time to Philadelphia nonprofit hospitals—all of these phenomena played against the backdrop of this faltering public hospital, which loomed large in the public consciousness as its failing became a highly public matter, the subject of multiple tabloid exposés. Within the context of these failures, and on the pages of the Philadelphia newspapers, a public debate raged over the life, circumstances, and (ultimate) fate of PGH.

What remains today of the Philadelphia General Hospital physical plant, is one small building used as an outpatient mental health facility and a brick and wrought-iron fence that serves as an entrance point to the Children's Hospital of Philadelphia (CHOP), and the research complex of CHOP and the University of Pennsylvania (PENN). What remains of the spirit of PGH is a noble tradition and aspiration, neither fully realized, nor fully extinguished.

1

Ascent and Aspiration: Early Development of Public Hospitals in America

Historical, Political, and Philosophical Underpinnings

In his treatise *On Liberty*, John Stuart Mill outlined the basis for a moral obligation to benevolence in civil society when he wrote:

> There are [also] many positive acts for the benefit of others, which he may rightfully be compelled to perform. . . .in any [other] joint work necessary to the interest of society of which he enjoys protection; and to perform certain acts of beneficence, such as saving a fellow creature's life, or interposing to protect the defenseless against ill usage, things which whenever it is obviously a man's duty to do, he may rightfully be made responsible to society for not doing. A person may cause evil to others not only by his action, but by his inaction, and in either case, is justly accountable to them for the injury.[1]

In 1859, when Mill published *On Liberty*, almshouses and dispensaries were the institutionalized form of benevolence for the sick and the poor in Europe and America.[2] The emergence of hospitals as agencies for caring and curing developed slowly from colonial America into the pre-Civil War period.[3] Predicated on European models of

1

benevolence and emerging notions of the "worthy poor," the sick, destitute, mentally ill, aged, and the infirm were often grouped together
within these early institutions. A later British model, as it found
expression on American shores, provided for the creation of voluntary
hospitals in addition to almshouses.[4] Almshouses, also called work
houses, were avoided by all but the most destitute. Often, common
criminals and debtors were required to provide care to those relegated
to these unfortunate places. In an effort to prevent the expansion of
appropriated funds from state coffers, the provisional government
intended that those in need should only get assistance in limited circumstances. They hoped that the stigma of the almshouse would cause
the needy to treat this as a last resort.

At this time, America was preoccupied with the nation-wrench-
ing events of the Civil War. But in the post-Civil War period of 1877 to
1920, the nation "moved rapidly from social simplicity to social complexity."[5] Isolated communities were replaced by one interdependent
nation, and provincial forms of social interaction assumed a more
cosmopolitan style and pattern. This trend toward interdependency
set the stage for new levels of bureaucracy, efficiency, and complexity
that are the hallmarks of 20th-century government programs.[6]

Differentiation in Health Care and Its Impact

Patterns of differentiation, which served as the constructs of the
emerging health care system, found expression in a variety of important venues:[7] in hospitals, which began to establish still-identifiable
frameworks; in medical practice, which gave rise to formalization in
medical education and specialization; in nursing practice with the
establishment of the training schools for nurses, including the school
founded by Alice Fisher at Philadelphia Hospital, which contributed to
the professionalization of the discipline of nursing; and in the group-
ing of patients for purposes of care delivery by establishing guidelines
that separated patients into categories such as sex, age, and types of illness and needs, further differentiating notions of care and cure.

Differentiation of Hospitals
The development of voluntary hospitals, with the concurrent development of public hospitals evolving from the almshouse/dispensary

models, was important in creating the framework of what is now regarded as the hospital system. Voluntary hospitals were frequently founded by various ethnic and religious groups and defined the earliest notions of a two-tier health care system: that which was dependent on charity (public), and that which was dependent on other mixes of private financing and the goodwill and philanthropy of others within a defined community of which one was a member (voluntary). These voluntary hospitals are the precursor institutions to non-profit hospitals as we know them today.

Differentiation in the Practice of Medicine

Throughout colonial America, the education of physicians and the practice of medicine were in their infancy. Medicine, loosely defined into four categories—medical treatment, surgery, pharmacy, and midwifery—was the basis of practice and often predicated on European education.[8] In the post-Revolutionary period, there was increasing emphasis on the establishment of American-based medical education. The emerging frameworks included privately run proprietary schools and university based schools. These programs consisted of classroom lectures and an apprenticeship with an established physician. The quality of the proprietary programs varied and was regarded by many to be inferior to their European counterparts.

The competing philosophy, advanced by the more elite group of physicians, sought to standardize and license medical education. These controversies, and the resulting political and turf battles, continued over many decades.[9] After the Civil War, there was an increasing interest in specialization. Physicians distanced themselves from the practice of pharmacy, leading to the emergence of druggists as a trade and the founding of the discipline of pharmacy.[10]

Differentiation in Nursing and Medical Practice at Philadelphia Hospital

The Era of Fisher and Osler at Old Blockley

The foundation of Philadelphia Hospital as a scientific and professional institution was laid in the years 1884 to 1888. In 1884, Alice Fisher and William Osler arrived in Philadelphia, she from England, he from Canada. The coincidence of their arrival heralded major developments in the emerging disciplines of nursing and medicine, respectively.[11]

Alice Fisher, a protégé of Florence Nightingale, was invited into service by two of Philadelphia's most prominent citizens, Anthony Drexel and George Childs, for the purpose of developing a professional training school for nurses. The search for a suitable candidate from the city or region had been ongoing for some time without success. Fisher had an established reputation for her work in England, where she served as superintendent of the General Hospital of Birmingham.[12] The intent of the hospital's new Board of Guardians for creating Fisher's role was to serve as a cornerstone in a reform movement, spurred in part by the response to corruption and malfeasance that was widely publicized in 1881.[13] The new board, convinced that improvement and professionalization of nursing would elevate the level and quality of care, engaged Fisher for the task. Edith Horner, who had served with Fisher in several important roles in England, accompanied her to assist in the development of the new school. In the first Duty Register of the training school for nursing, the earliest entries[14] demonstrate that Fisher sought quickly to establish order and hierarchy on the wards by listing the staff on duty and using the term "head nurse" to define the supervisory role assigned to each unit.[15]

Alice Fisher was the daughter of a well-educated and well-placed family. Her father, Head Master of Eton College, was nursed from illness to health by his daughter. This inspired Fisher in her early life to undertake nursing. She pursued her profession at St. Thomas Training School in London, and was one of its earliest graduates. After graduation, she worked at the Royal Infirmary of Edinburgh and later in the Fever Hospital in New Castle. She served as superintendent of the Adinbroke Hospital in Cambridge, then as superintendent in Birmingham. From there, she set sail for Philadelphia on September 9, 1884.[16]

While at sea, Alice Fisher became acquainted with Mrs. Henry Fisher of Jenkintown, who was part of a group of influential women from the Philadelphia area. During their voyage, Alice Fisher used the time to engage these women of standing in her aspirations for her work. By the time they disembarked in Philadelphia, Alice Fisher's new friends became philanthropic supporters, raising money and securing food, clothing, and other necessities for the hospital and the nurses under her care and supervision.[17]

As she embarked on the work ahead of her, Alice Fisher faced significant challenges that slowed and stymied reform. Perception of her as an outsider also added to local suspicions. She faced these and a multitude of other obstacles with equanimity. In an address to the graduating class of the Training School for Nurses in 1893, Dr. J. William White, a friend and supporter of Fisher, delivered a speech in which he posthumously revered her, speaking of

> . . . the skill, energy, and perseverance with which. . . she overcame the obstacles that custom fortified by ignorance or stupidity on the one hand and by malice or absolute dishonesty on the other, placed in her way. One by one, the barriers thus erected disappeared before her persistent protests or persuasive elegance. . . mortality in the hospital decreased so that it became apparent—and demonstrable—that many lives were being saved through her labors.[18]

White also described Fisher as having "an attractive and winning personality"[19] and declared that "Bravery, too, was among her virtues, having not been disturbed by threats against her life" (being blown up with dynamite), or facing a malignant outbreak of typhoid in Plymouth, Pennsylvania, where she went to care for the ill for two months.[20]

Alice Fisher spent the last four years of her life at Old Blockley, building a legacy of professional nursing care for the patients and staff at Philadelphia Hospital. In her last year, confined to a wheelchair, she continued to participate in the development and stabilization of the school of nursing, to which she was deeply committed. Under her leadership, nurses participated in lectures given by many eminent physicians of the day, in addition to her tutelage and that of Edith Horner. Physicians were required to write down their orders so that nurses could refer to them. New nurses, or probationers, were recruited and educated so that they were literate enough to read them. The rigorous schedules and intense supervision by Fisher and Horner infused the hospital with a new culture that bespoke a focus on civility, decency, and the application of scientific principles in the care of patients.

It has been speculated that the intensity with which Alice Fisher pursued her work contributed to her ill health and hastened the end of her life. Dr. White believed that Alice Fisher literally worked herself to death. She knew she had a heart condition, but despite his medical advice, insisted on continuing her vocation until her death on June 3, 1888. Fisher was visited on the day of her death by her friend and colleague, William Osler, who wrote in his journal that day, "I have just left the deathbed of Miss Fisher, a sweet blessed character whose influence on others has been great in. . . " The entry trailed off. Osler's colleague and friend Henry Cushing later speculated that Osler was overcome with grief, unable to complete his thoughts on paper.[21] Osler and White served as pallbearers for Alice Fisher's funeral, thus marking the end of her remarkable career at Old Blockley. Less than a year later William Osler himself would leave Philadelphia Hospital.

Dr. William Osler came to Philadelphia Hospital in 1884, with his distinguished career well underway, to serve as professor of clinical medicine at the University of Pennsylvania. He was extensively educated, receiving multiple degrees from major universities in Canada, England, Berlin, and Vienna. He also attended Yale, Harvard, and Johns Hopkins. Osler became well known for a meticulous research style that found expression in postmortem examinations. During his time at Philadelphia Hospital, he conducted vast numbers of thoroughly documented postmortem exams, often of patients he had seen in the wards, adding congruence to his lived observations.[22] He established the "Green Room," also known as the "Post Room," where autopsies were conducted and medical students educated. To accommodate the large number of students seeking to observe Osler's work, a hole was cut into the ceiling so that the second floor of the building could be used by additional students watching from above.[23]

Like Fisher, Osler was beloved by his students and colleagues. He saw patients in his private offices on South 15th Street, near Chestnut,[24] and routinely welcomed all students. His research methods were somewhat controversial. At a time when microscopes were rarely used in clinical practice, Osler brought his microscope to the hospital and examined the blood of any number of patients, seeking to make or confirm a diagnosis, especially of malaria or other suspected parasitic diseases. He sought to replicate the earlier discovery of Charles Louis Laveran that had been met with widespread skepticism in the international medical community. While few other physicians were impressed, Osler pursued the parasitic theory Laveran had advanced. Using his microscope, he invented a method to count blood corpuscles.[25]

Osler left Philadelphia to accept a post at the new Johns Hopkins University Hospital in Baltimore to serve as professor of medicine and physician-in-chief.[26] Over the years, he continued to collaborate and correspond with many of his former students and colleagues who gave him substantial credit for their accomplishments, having been educated and trained by him.[27]

At the time of his death, William Osler was probably the most renowned physician in the world, leaving a significant body of work that spanned several decades and continents. While Osler was best known for his work in the discovery of typhoid and malaria and had conducted extensive studies on smallpox at McGill University in Canada before his arrival in Philadelphia, he was engaged in multiple areas of research due to a diverse clinical practice and a fertile intellectual curiosity. During his time at the Philadelphia Hospital, he studied and lectured on typhoid, Jacksonian epilepsy, childhood cerebral palsies, infantile paralysis, differential diagnosis of smallpox versus varicella, cirrhosis of the liver in children and adults, gallstones, pernicious anemia, Bright's disease, Weil's disease, Hodgkin's disease, pneumonia, gastric and duodenal ulcers, spina bifida, and literally hundreds of other clinical topics.[28]

Specialization in Medical Practice at Philadelphia Hospital

From 1877 to 1904, Philadelphia Hospital established multiple specialty departments.[29] In each of these departments, in addition to treating patients, the physicians, clinicians, and scientists were generating significant volumes of early scholarly publications. In the first volume of *Philadelphia Hospital Reports*,[30] a summary of academic and clinical work in 1890, there were dozens of report submissions, including "Pyo-hydronephrosis caused by pyelitis and urethritis of gonococcal origin," "Scurvy," "Puerperal septicemia simulating typhoid fever," "The practical value of modern methods of antisepsis in the care of infants," "The therapeutic uses of the nitrites," "A study of the Bacillus subtilis," and "Erysipelas of the eyelids spreading extensively to the face and scalp." The fourth volume, published in 1893, included a report entitled "Eighty-six successful cataract operations in the Philadelphia Hospital," as well as other ophthalmologic reports on removal of an epithelioma and successful blepharoplasty. These reports illuminate the level of activity in the newly specialized department of ophthalmology. Other reports included one by Dr. Mills on syphilis of the nervous system and a report by Dr. Kluttz of a case of double parotitis, along with many other clinical renderings, further defining the emerging scientific rigor with which the Philadelphia Hospital's medical staff were pursuing their knowledge and practice goals.[31]

In 1900, Philadelphia Hospital enjoyed the prestige of another significant development. Dr. Daniel Hughes, the chief resident physician, assisted by Dr. Charles Leonard, a pioneer in the field on staff at the time as an anesthetist, established the Roentgen Laboratory.[32] "Roentgens" and their potential clinical applications had been discovered only a few years earlier in 1895 by German physics professor Wilhelm Roentgen. In less than two years after the new department had been established, more than 800 Roentgen method examinations had been completed, including the second diagnosis ever made of a brain tumor by this method. Treatments for cancer and skin diseases followed. In 1921, the City of Philadelphia purchased 2 grams of radium for $157,000, the first city in the United States to do so, in an effort to make free treatment available for cancer patients and those requiring radiation therapy for other illnesses. Later, the hospital opened a separate radiological department, further catalyzing scientific advances.[33]

History of Philadelphia General Hospital

The Philadelphia General Hospital that closed its doors in 1977 was actually the third incarnation of previous embodiments of public altruism in Philadelphia dating back to the 1700s.[34] The early predecessors included an almshouse at 4th and Spruce Streets, and a later, larger version at 10th and Spruce Streets. In 1828, the Board of Trustees, responding to an expansion of the city's boundaries, purchased 187 acres in the township of Blockley upon which they would build the Almshouse, Hospital, House of Employment, and Children's Asylum.[35] As the focus of the institution continued to refine itself, the official name was changed to The Philadelphia Hospital in 1835.

In the early to mid-19th century, the hospital was dominated by political patronage. A newspaper account quoted Dr. H.G. Woods, who, when describing the hospital leadership, characterized them as the "Board of Buzzards."[36] Even though the early medical care was donated by many of the most prominent physicians of the time, the pervasive squalor was unprecedented and unrelenting. These poor conditions continued until the introduction of formalized nursing care in 1885. This new nursing order, crafted by Alice Fisher, gave rise to a reputation of excellence for Philadelphia Hospital and the city, in the practice of nursing and medicine.[37]

In 1887, the Pennsylvania legislature passed the Bullit Bill, which restructured many city governmental functions and created the Civil Service Commission.[38] This act was an attempt to depoliticize the functions of government and to ensure that talented, devoted citizens were placed into positions of public service and public trust. Hence, the newly constituted Commission made all subsequent leadership appointments, including the successor to Alice Fisher, Chief Nurse Marion Smith, who took the first Civil Service Exam.[39]

In 1902, the hospital's official name became The Philadelphia General Hospital, and the Bullit Act was amended to create the Department of Public Health and Charities. The post of Public Health Director was created and the hospital placed under his control. With a city charter change in 1920, the care for the mentally ill was moved from PGH to the new facilities of Byberry and for the well-poor to Holmesberg, while the Department of Public Health and the Department of Welfare developed separate roles under their newly created separate banners.[40] Once again PGH was transformed, this time into a large municipal hospital focused on the medical needs of its citizens, poor and otherwise. The change in venue contributed to the public perception, intentionally fostered by the governing board and leading physicians, that the focus of the institution was care of the sick, emphasizing a decided break with the past. This shift was important in order to establish PGH as a center for medical care and excellence and to remove the social stigma associated with care of the indigent and the insane. In 1920, PGH superintendent Dr. Joseph Doane appealed to the citizens to recognize this. By 1924, it appeared that the citizenry had heeded his call, as PGH began to attract paying patients in numbers that began to generate significant revenue.[41] Within this context, the reputation of PGH developed.

Notes

1. John Stuart Mill, "On Liberty," in *The World's Greatest Thinkers: Man and State, Political Philosophers*, eds. Saxe Commins and Robert N. Linscott (New York: Random House, 1947), 146.

2. Charles E. Rosenberg, "Social Class and Medical Care in 19th-Century America: The Rise and Fall of the Dispensary," in *Sickness and Health in America: Readings in the History of Medicine and Public Health*, eds. Judith Walzer Leavitt and Ronald L. Numbers, 3rd ed. (Madison: University of Wisconsin Press, 1997), 309-322.

3. See Harry F. Dowling, *City Hospitals: The Undercare of the Underprivileged* (Cambridge, MA: Harvard University Press, 1982), 9-13; Charles E. Rosenberg, "Community and Communities: The Evolution of the American Hospital," in *The American General Hospital: Communities and Social Contexts*, eds. Diana E. Long and Janet Golden (Ithaca, NY: Cornell University Press, 1989), 3-20; Rosemary Stevens, *American Medicine and the Public Interest* (New Haven, CT: Yale University Press, 1976), 9-54.

4. Dowling, 9-10.

5. S. Skowronek, *Building a New American State: The Expansion of National Administrative Capacities, 1877-1920* (New York: Cambridge University Press, 1982), 11-12.

6. Ibid., especially chapters 3, 5, 6, and 8.

7. See Charles E. Rosenberg, *Explaining Epidemics and Other Studies in the History of Medicine* (Cambridge, UK: Cambridge University Press, 1992), chapter 19 for extensive discussion on differentiation and the emergence of early health care system structure.

8. Stevens, 20, as well as chapters 1-3.

9. Ibid., 20-30.

10. Ibid., 31. Specialized pharmacy schools were founded in the early 1800's in Philadelphia, New York, and Chicago.

11. For brief summaries of Osler and Fisher, see John Welsh Croskey, *History of Blockley* (Philadelphia: F.A. Davis, 1929), 469-470; Charles K. Mills, "The Philadelphia Almshouse and Philadelphia Hospital from 1854 to 1908," in *The History of Blockley*, ed. John Welsh Croskey (Philadelphia: F.A. Davis, 1929), 91-92. Also see S.A. Stachniewicz, and J.K. Axelrod, *The Double Frill: The History of the Philadelphia General Hospital and the School of Nursing* (Philadelphia: George F. Stickley, 1978), 31, for more background on Alice Fisher and the founding of the School of Nursing.

12. Lillian Clayton, "School of Nursing," in *The History of Blockley*, ed. John Welsh Croskey (Philadelphia: F.A. Davis, 1929), 146-148.

13. Mills, 90-92.

14. The original duty register instituted by Fisher and Horner is part of the College of Physicians' archival collection of PGH. The register is bound in leather and engraved with the title Philadelphia Hospital and the year 1885. Since Fisher arrived in Philadelphia within weeks of commencing her work, it is likely that she had the duty register created in England before her arrival, predicated on her existing practices and inclinations.

15. Ibid. See the ward designations and the staff assignments entered into the register. The wards were delineated as men's surgical, women's surgical, men's medicine, women's medicine, men's nerves, women's nerves, obstetrics, and pavilions.

16. Clayton, 146-148.

17. Ibid., 147-148.

18. J. William White, "Alice Fisher," in *Philadelphia Hospital Reports*, eds. C.K. Mills and James W. Walk, Volume II (Philadelphia: J.B. Lippincott, 1893), 14.

19. Ibid., 14.

20. Ibid.

21. Stachniewicz and Axelrod, 31.

22. See *Sir William Osler Memorial Volume, Appreciations and Reminiscences*, ed. Maude Abbott (privately issued at 836 University Street, Montreal, Canada), Second Impression, 1927. See especially the extensive annotation of his work by time period, institution, and category in the College of Physicians' Osler collection.

23. For anecdotal accounts of Osler's medical school teaching, see the speeches of his former students in the Osler Memorial Committee papers, Box 1, folder series 1.2, May 1940, "Osler/attended to" correspondence, the College of Physicians' Osler collection.

24. This was revealed on page 1 in a draft speech to be given by a former student/resident, Dr. Joseph McFarland, at the dedication of the Osler Memorial. McFarland was a resident under Osler at the Philadelphia Hospital in 1889. See the Osler Memorial Committee papers, Box 1, folder series 1.2, May 1940, "Osler/attended to" correspondence, May 1940, the College of Physicians' Osler collection.

25. Ibid.

26. Croskey, 470.

27. See all of the speeches from the Osler Memorial dedication in the Osler Memorial Committee papers, including J. McFarland, W.G. McCallum, John Bower, William Hughes, and A.A. Eshner, Box 1, folder series 1.2, May 1940, "Osler/attended to" correspondence. Also see the speeches of Robert Hunter, Box 4, folder series 4.2, the College of Physicians' Osler collection.

28. Croskey, 517-531.

29. In 1877, the neurological department, or Nervous Wards, for men and women was established, along with departments in ophthalmology and dermatology. In 1885, the training school for nurses opened. In 1889, the bacteriological department was established; in 1890, the laryngological department, and in 1892, the isolation department. In 1900, the departments of pediatrics and orthopedics, and the first Roentgen laboratory for diagnosis and treatment were opened. In 1901 and 1903, the oral surgery department and the clinical laboratory opened, respectively. And in 1904, the tuberculosis department and the venereal and genito-urinary departments were established. Mills, 85. For more background on medical specialization, see Stevens, chapters 1, 2, and 3.

30. This first volume was edited by Dr. Charles Mills and Dr. James Walk, and was printed in Philadelphia by J.B. Lippincott in 1890. In the preface, it reads: "The history and reminiscences of every great charitable institution like the Philadelphia Almshouse and Hospital should, moreover, be placed upon the record for the guidance and instruction of present and future generations." (v)

31. *Philadelphia Hospital Reports*, eds. Roland G. Curtin and Daniel Hughes (Philadelphia: J.B. Lippincott, 1900), the College of Physicians' PGH collection.

32. Mills, 95-96.

33. Ibid.

34. See Charles M. Rosenberg, *The Care of Strangers: The Rise of America's Hospital System* (Baltimore: The Johns Hopkins University Press, 1987), 27-39, 322-329.

35. Stachniewicz and Axelrod, 9-11.

36. J. Chalmers Da Costa, "The Old Blockley Hospital: Its Characters and Characteristics," in *The History of Blockley*, ed. John Welsh Croskey (Philadelphia: F.A. Davis, 1929), 135.

37. See Rosenberg, *The Care of Strangers*, 8-9; Stachniewicz and Axelrod, 9-32; Susan M. Reverby, *Ordered to Care: The Dilemma of American Nursing, 1850-1945* (New York: Cambridge University Press, 1987).

38. Stachniewicz and Axelrod, 11.

39. Ibid.

40. Mayor's Committee on Municipal Health Services, *Report of the Mayor's Committee on Municipal Health Services* (Philadelphia: Mayor's Committee on Municipal Health Services, February 1970).

41. Stachniewicz and Axelrod, 12. In 1924, PGH recorded revenues of more than $100,000 from paying patients.

2

Hill-Burton, Medicare, and Medicaid: The Politics, Policies, and Impact of Federal Health Care Expansion

Throughout the development of modern democracy and American government, questions of obligation to those less fortunate have occupied philosophical, ideological, and political dialogues, and catalyzed public policy debates.[1] Rooted in 18th- and early 19th-century notions of benevolence, civil society's grappling with the complexities of caring for its sick and dependent found expression across the decades in social, civic, legislative, and bureaucratic actions and trends.

The emergence of a 20th-century system of health care delivery and payment was largely predicated on the development and implementation of three landmark pieces of legislation: Hill-Burton, first enacted under President Truman, with subsequent amendments and expansions under Eisenhower, Kennedy, and Johnson; and the passage of Medicare and Medicaid, under President Johnson, which were the centerpieces of his Great Society antipoverty program. The passage and implementation of these pieces of legislation signaled a shift in the ideological underpinnings for care of the poor, the infirm, and the aged across racial lines. Examination of the impact of these key pieces of legislation yields an expansive backdrop against which to view the dynamics of large-scale health care delivery trends. This analysis brings into perspective the significance of these policy developments and informs, from a historical point of view, the sweeping changes that preceded and followed.

Moving Hospitals Toward Center Stage in Health Care Delivery

In the late 19th and early 20th centuries, boards of trustees of hospitals attempted to increase hospital usage by the middle-class, who were previously cared for at home.[2] Since many hospitals still carried the stigma from their earlier almshouse days, in which only the poor, destitute, and undesirables were cared for within the walls of the institution, hospital beds were often empty.

The stigma was a subject of debate and discussion by the urban elite. At the opening of the Boston City Hospital in the 1870's, its president, Thomas Amory Jr., described a recent attempt by a former Massachusetts governor to assist in the cause when he, having been injured and despite having had the means to employ a private physician in his home, was taken to the hospital. Amory concluded his remarks by touching on another reason that individuals continued to decline a hospital stay, saying that he did not believe that those better off would willingly go to the hospital ". . . among strangers to be cured."[3] Clearly, the effort of hospital leadership to persuade citizens that hospitals were the best means toward health and recovery was not an easy task.

Due to the difficulty in establishing critical mass by increasing admissions, managing the upkeep of a hospital with insufficient revenue streams was problematic for the trustees trying to lead and sustain these early institutions. In a World War I–era edition of the journal *Hospital Management*, an advertisement demonstrated the importance of "selling" the community on the idea that they, as patients, could receive better care in the hospital, as opposed to home, under the treatment of a private physician.[4] This advertising approach suggested they had a patriotic duty to do so.

Three central themes emerged for the trustees and administrators of these early 20th-century institutions: the importance of having a hospital in one's community; the significance of how a hospital defines its mission; and a sense that increasing the scale of the hospital was the only way to finance a "saleable" operation. These leaders recognized that they needed to consider alternative routes of appeal to increase usage by the middle class and wealthy patients. Fortunately, other factors contributed to create dynamic shifts in the marketplace.

The Advent of Health Insurance

In the late 1950's and throughout the decade of the 1960's, employer-based, third-party health insurance became a dominant factor in the financing of hospital-based care. In 1951, the Commission on the Financing of Hospital Care was established as an independent, non-governmental agency. The establishment of this commission followed the work of the Commission on Hospital Care, discussed later, which issued its report in 1947. The extensive report, led by the American Hospital Association and other key constituencies, framed out 181 principles and recommendations and sought to balance need, opportunity, financing, and capital expansion.[5] The successor three-volume report, generated after two years of study by the Commission on the Financing of Hospital Care, offers a comprehensive review of the problems and accomplishments of the post–World War II health care system. Most notably, it delineated the populations that were covered and not covered by prepaid insurance plans. Based on data gleaned from the commission, 87 percent of all Americans were insured at some level for hospital care via employment, principally though a Blue Cross plan.[6] By 1960, 63 percent of all nongovernmental expenditures (beyond individual and group coverage) on hospital services were covered by Blue Cross plans, or some other insurance plan.[7]

A driver in the expansion of employer-based health insurance was the emergence of unions as agents of collective bargaining. After World War II, wage increases were restricted. A series of successful legal challenges led to health care benefits becoming an automatic part and focus of collective bargaining. Under these conditions, unions recognized that employer-based, employer-paid health insurance was of central importance to their members.[8] Once unions gained standing after the passage of the Wagner Act, part of the New Deal programs under President Roosevelt, expanded benefit plans quickly followed.[9] The phenomenon of employer-based insurance achieved two important side benefits for hospitals: first, employee-based benefits were employer-subsidized, thus expanding the pool of covered lives; second, the use of wage- or work-related insurance provided structured coverage toward the able-bodied, and away from the more high-intensity users, including the aged and the indigent.

Most importantly, the Commission on Hospital Financing focused on the demographic gaps in health insurance coverage. Significant gaps were noted in the retired aged, the unemployed, and in low-income families. The analysis of this issue, which clearly identified the groups that, a decade later, would be the beneficiaries of Medicare and Medicaid, concluded by saying: "Adequate financing of hospital care in communities throughout the nation cannot be achieved until a more orderly plan has been instituted for financing the care of the non-wage and low income groups."[10]

Precedents to Hill-Burton

The passage of the Lanham Act and the creation of the Commission on Hospital Care were two important events that preceded the introduction and passage of Hill-Burton.[11] The Lanham Act, introduced by Congressman Fritz Lanham of Texas, passed in 1941. Implemented through 1943, this legislation established an important precedent, providing federal funding to nonprofit hospitals that would be controlled by the community. This war-related public works project was a key driver in the notion that the federal government can and should lead the way for redefining access to capital financing and enabling communities to assume responsibility for local development and growth in matters of national importance. From 1941 to 1946, 874 hospital construction projects were completed.[12]

The second important precedent to Hill-Burton was the work of the Commission on Hospital Care. The Commission, a cross-disciplinary effort jointly backed and administered by the American Hospital Association, the U.S. Public Health Service, and the Kellogg Foundation, issued its first report in 1947 after two years of deliberation.[13] The Commission's focus was to encourage and assist the states to evaluate the need for hospital expansion and modernization. It created working groups to study these areas with the charge to develop quantitative guidelines. Once established, these guidelines would serve as the basis for a state-by-state blueprint. The expectation was that each state, in concert with the federal government, would use this blueprint to pursue a cogent plan for hospital expansion and growth. Following the work of this commission was a sequel, the Commission on the Financing of Hospital Care. This entity, similarly established as a quasi-governmental organization, created work groups among key constituencies to develop an understanding of the options for financing health care delivery and made extensive recommendations for establishing a network to fund this system.[14] These extensive studies served as a base of information for the Great Society programs that would follow.

Expansion of the Health Care System and Hill-Burton

President Roosevelt first proposed legislation to fund construction of rural hospitals in 1940. This proposal came on the heels of federally funded programs, first implemented during the Depression, that provided varying levels of federal support. These federal monies also spurred state funding that was driven, in large part, by the passage of the Social Security Act of 1935. The introduction of the bill was preceded by the dramatic fiscal turmoil of the Depression, which adversely affected the voluntary hospital sector. While Roosevelt's proposal passed the Senate with bipartisan support, it failed in the House. In 1946, when Hill-Burton was passed, it was a more expansive bill than the one introduced by Roosevelt's allies in the Senate. Sponsored by Senator Lister Hill of Alabama, a Republican, and Senator Harold Burton of Ohio, a Democrat, this bill addressed construction of voluntary hospitals and nonprofit facilities in both urban and rural settings.

The revised bipartisan bill represented an expansion across interest groups and was amended to appeal to members of Congress who represented urban districts. This political strategy, combined with the softening of opposition from physician groups, made passage of Hill-Burton possible. Most importantly, it was proposed in the immediate postwar period when the United States was facing dramatic drops in production in a variety of markets.

In a cabinet meeting with President Truman in 1945, Secretary of Commerce Henry Wallace estimated that the Gross National Product (GNP) would decrease by $40 billion, including $20 billion in lost wages, and result in the unemployment of eight million Americans.

This decline would amount to a functional return to the Great Depression. Economic stimulus supported by federal public works projects would be key in preventing a national postwar fiscal disaster.[15] These phenomena contributed mightily to the need to refocus the national economy. In a radio broadcast, President Truman stated, "Nineteen-hundred and forty-six is our year of decision. This year, we lay the foundation for our economic structure which will have to serve for generations."[16]

The Politics of Hill-Burton Passage

The principal leading the charge for public financing of hospitals was George Bugbee, the executive director of the American Hospital Association, a registered Washington lobbyist, and an associate of Senator Harold Burton from Ohio.[17] Burton agreed to introduce the bill, contingent on Senator Taft's approval. Taft, though not in favor of national health insurance of any kind but needing a health care bill for his presidential platform, agreed. Senator Hill was recruited to ensure bipartisan support, and Hill-Burton was introduced in 1945.[18]

The Hospital Survey and Construction Act, better known as Hill-Burton, was signed into law by President Truman the following year. The act was a centerpiece and driving force for postwar hospital construction and was "the most important piece of legislation in the postwar decade."[19] It was also the central driver for the development of academic medical centers to meet increased demand for health care service delivery.[20] Hill-Burton gave an economic boost to the country at a critical time, spurring new construction and modernization projects across America, remodeling and expanding outdated facilities, and redefining the landscape of health care delivery. The implementation resulted in dramatic expansions within the hospital sector, increasing the total number of hospitals from 785 in 1946 to 1,704 in 1970.[21] By 1980, there were 4,090 hospitals participating in the Hill-Burton program.[22]

A key component of Hill-Burton initially was its capacity to provide outright grants for hospital infrastructure construction. The law required that hospitals receiving funds under the program provide uncompensated care for 20 years in an amount matching either 3 percent of its annual operating costs or 10 percent of the total federal assistance received, whichever was less. Each hospital could set its own eligibility requirements, which ranged between 100 and 200 percent of the federal poverty level.[23] Later the law was amended to provide tax-exempt financing through qualified state agencies. States were permitted to offer federally matched financing for large-scale construction projects using these quasi-governmental agencies or authorities. These authorities were often set up by local governments, counties, or municipalities, with enacting legislation from state government, and gave local elected and appointed officials and hospital boards and executives more access and control of tax-exempt, long-term bonds. Local leadership was thus enabled to drive local expansion and planning.[24]

Hill-Burton was not only important for what it did in its first incarnation, but also for what followed. The program was extended over the next two decades to include construction of nursing homes and of diagnostic, rehabilitation, and treatment centers (1954); long-term loans (1958); out-of-hospital community facilities (1961); and hospital modernization (1964).[25]

In 1964, with the passage of the Civil Rights Act, Hill-Burton had additional impact on hospitals. It eliminated the "separate but equal" policy, thus affecting the Title III, VI, and VIII federal programs. The Civil Rights Act prohibited discrimination in any programs receiving federal assistance, including public building projects, job training, and education. It provided for more extensive surveillance to ensure compliance and made violators subject to suit by the United States Attorney General, with attendant penalties, including interruption of federal funding. It also established the Equal Employment Opportunity Commission (EEOC), which was empowered to investigate possible racial discrimination and provide support should a federal lawsuit ensue.[26] Ultimately, this had significant impact on PGH, since Philadelphia hospitals were now required to accept African-American patients. It would only be a matter of time until non-Caucasian patients would exercise their right to choose their health care provider.

The War on Poverty and the Advent of Medicare and Medicaid

In his ground-breaking book, *The Other America*, published in 1962, Michael Harrington detailed the origins and impact of poverty in Appalachia, bringing the shadowy outlines of the face of rural American poverty into view.[27] The Harrington book, combined with an essay written for the *New Yorker* by Dwight MacDonald on the invisible poor, moved then-President John F. Kennedy toward the development of a plan, to be implemented after his reelection in 1964, that would break the intractable cycle of poverty described by Harrington and MacDonald. The full development of the plan would be preceded by an extensive visit to poverty-stricken areas of America that had been largely invisible to the average American. Kennedy and his advisors would devote two to three full presidential days to the trip. They believed that when average Americans saw the level of suffering within their own borders, they would be moved by compassion to support the President's program. But Kennedy understood that in order to advance a large-scale social program, he would have to do something that helped the middle class as well as the poor. "Let's make clear," he argued, "that we're doing something for the middle-income man in the suburbs as well."[28]

Kennedy's intent was to attack American poverty by developing a coordinated set of programs. He sent an early signal in a 1961 speech to Congress by strongly endorsing hospital insurance for the aged through Social Security.[29] On the eve of his assassination, John Kennedy was poised and determined to give the American people a clear view of the pain of poverty in America, and the opportunity to address it in expansive new programs to care for the aged and the indigent. After his death, his brother Robert found a sheet of paper with notes the President had written in his last cabinet meeting. The word "poverty" was written repeatedly and circled. Robert Kennedy had that piece of paper framed and hung in his office.[30]

It was JFK's successor, Lyndon Johnson, and his own brother[31] who brought the poverty of Appalachia into the living rooms of America during their highly publicized excursions into the heartland of America's silent poor.[32] President Johnson picked up the gauntlet that JFK, fate, and circumstance had thrown down. In his first State of the Union Address, Johnson declared "an unconditional war on poverty."[33] The first wave of his legislative agenda was outlined in the 1964 Economic Opportunity Act.[34]

The Politics of Poverty

President Kennedy rightly understood the political utility and importance of linking a poverty program with a benefit for middle-class

Americans.[35] But Lyndon Johnson, who had great faith in his capabilities as a legislative tactician and an absolute focus on securing his place in history while ensuring his political viability and reelection, had much grander objectives. During his presidency, the war on poverty took on almost mythic proportions as Johnson skillfully tied it to the program of the assassinated President,[36] and, by extension, the civil rights movement, health care for the aged, and other "Great Society" antipoverty programs.[37] Johnson, in part with an eye toward solidifying his political base and reelection and toward a lasting legacy, made the passage of Medicare and Medicaid central to his domestic program. The connection to the murdered president made it almost impossible for Congress to deny Johnson success in his pursuit of a legislative victory.[38] Johnson knew that passage of these keystone pieces of legislation would ensure his place in history, saying, "Kennedy would live on forever, and so would I."[39]

There were clearly sentiments that could be tapped among the populace to advance the late President's agenda. But there was still a great deal of difficulty in moving this massive program through Congress. President Johnson's antipoverty bill was sent to Congress on March 16, 1964, with an appropriations request of $962.5 million.

The scope and grandiosity of the Johnson legislative agenda was stunning. By the summer of 1965, the President signed multiple bills he had championed, and still had other major pieces of legislation in the pipeline.[40] In his second year as President, Johnson dominated his old stomping ground of the Congress. More so than any other President, the Congressional agenda was his agenda. Given an unprecedented mandate and an overwhelming majority in the House (295 Democrats), Johnson seemed unstoppable. In the Senate, of which he had been the most powerful and influential leader only a few years earlier, the men with whom he had served were still his friends and still held the reins of leadership.

LBJ and RFK: The Politics of Competition

One of the most difficult and complex political byplays, which had substantive impact on the quality of the legislation that passed, was the need for LBJ to dominate the arena. That meant giving no quarter, and no opportunity, to the brother and heir presumptive of his late predecessor. While Bobby Kennedy was an integral, even central figure in the development of these important policy initiatives in the Kennedy White House, during the Johnson heyday, he was the junior senator from New York. Johnson knew intuitively that Kennedy would someday seek the presidency. The only question for Johnson was whether he would be a successor or a challenger to Johnson himself. So, in his preemptive style, Johnson sought to show public deference and respect to the martyred President's brother. But behind closed doors, Johnson sought out every opportunity to marginalize Bobby Kennedy substantively and, by extension, politically.[41]

One of the consequences of Johnson's approach, and his competitiveness with Bobby Kennedy, was that the legislative agenda, originally formulated by John Kennedy with Bobby, was passed in less useful form than had that same legislation been developed in concert with Bobby. Since Bobby was more likely to be true to the spirit of the legislation his brother had conceived, the content would likely have been more focused, less expansive, and more substantively and operationally sound. But in order to participate at all, Senator Kennedy was forced to react legislatively by amendment.[42] As it was, the convolution associated with the passage of Medicare and Medicaid became a legendary case of Johnson, the master of the Senate, imposing his will regardless of the collateral damage to public policy. It produced what historian, and then White House aide, Doris Kearns Goodwin, called the "politics of haste," with success measured not in solving a problem, but in passing a law.[43]

Progress, Pitfalls, and a Three-Layer Cake

In 1960, the American appetite for federal help with medical care was growing. The Kerr-Mills Bill, passed that year, provided limited, means-tested benefits for a prescribed number of services, but reformers found this unacceptable. They sought an extension of Social Security benefits for all elderly, without the bureaucratic, burdensome, stigmatizing means tests that the states desired. In 1962, President Kennedy urged Congress to pass the King-Anderson Medicare Bill. It was more extensive than Kerr-Mills, included hospitalization and nursing home costs, but omitted surgical coverage and physician fees. It was defeated after a massive campaign by the American Medical Association, following similar efforts by the Kennedy administration.[44]

In 1964, Johnson began his campaign for Medicare, one of his "Big Four" proposals.[45] Using his still-significant relationships and leverage in the Senate, he engineered the attachment of an amendment for hospital care in a Social Security bill. However, the bill lost momentum in a conference committee. This was the first time any federal legislative body had attempted to pass a health care bill of this magnitude. The amendment gave Johnson the help he needed for a significant edge on an important issue in the 1964 election.

In another significant political development, the Ways and Means Committee, chaired by Wilbur Mills, an opponent of Medicare, changed composition. Added were two new Democratic members who supported Medicare.[46] Now a pro-Medicare majority sat on the committee that oversaw Social Security. Chairman Mills, lacking a majority of votes, would not be able to hold it back. With increasing clamor from voters, Mills, who had a good sense of shifting political tides, changed his position.

In March 1965, the Mills Bill passed the Ways and Means subcommittee. The bill, described by Johnson as "a three-layer cake,"[47] was structured to include three major provisions: hospital coverage via extension of Social Security; coverage of physician payments under a voluntary insurance program; and state-managed, means-tested support for the indigent, including welfare recipients, the disabled, the blind, the aged, and children of single parents. This last provision was intended to provide matching federal grants to states to fund the program.[48]

The Mills Bill passed the House soon after it emerged from committee with 313 votes in favor and 115 opposed. The bill went on to the Senate, where Johnson outmaneuvered his friend Senator Harry Byrd of Virginia, an opponent of Medicare. Johnson managed to get Byrd onto a television station, where he coaxed him on camera, to assert that these important hearings would be promptly arranged. The bill, shepherded and amended extensively by Senator Russell Long, passed the Senate, 68-21. Once in conference committee, Mills outmaneuvered Long, and managed to remove most of the Senate amendments. In June, both houses passed Mills' three-layer-cake bill.[49]

Passed in 1965, Medicare and Medicaid created significant, dedicated funding streams for low-income citizens and the aged to access health care. Medicare covered all persons over age 65 and disabled individuals regardless of age. Medicaid, a federal-state cost-sharing program, covered all who passed a means test to assess poverty level. For the first time, there were dedicated funds for care of the poor. The significance of this was multipronged. It created direct funding that could be recovered by hospitals providing care to the indigent. Previous to this, those who had no health care insurance either had to pay out of pocket for their care, or rely on services available from public hospitals, public clinics, or religious institutions that evidenced a charitable mission.

At the time of the passage of Medicare and Medicaid, 75 percent of the population was covered by private medical insurance. The remaining 25 percent was largely composed of the elderly, the poor, and the unemployed. These groups, previously without access, were brought into the health care system and dramatically increased their utilization of medical services. From 1965 to 1980, the number of admissions to nonfederal hospitals increased 50 percent. Those over age 65 were responsible for most of the increase. The liberal Medicare reimbursement policies influenced private insurers to increase their flexibility in payment for services, since government precedent for payment was setting new industry standards.[50]

The Politics of Race, Health Care Coverage, and Access

When the first version of Hill-Burton was passed in final form, it did not include any requirements that hospitals receiving Hill-Burton funds operate without regard to race, creed, or color. The bill, and its political configuration, was another example of the continuing battle lines drawn in the Congress over race. In fact, the Senate rejected an amendment that would have included antidiscrimination provisions.

"States' rights" in implementation were urged by one of the co-sponsors of the bill, Senator Lister Hill of Alabama, as he worked to exclude the antidiscrimination provision. Hill asserted that it might be best to leave the details to the states, alluding to states' rights as the standard for implementation. But states' rights had, in the post-Civil War period, become one of the last verbal vestiges of organized discrimination against blacks.[51] It served as a code expression, indicating that the racial sensitivities of the white majority in the states were not to be interfered with, and that states were to be left to their own political inclinations.[52] A politically important Southern Democrat, Hill was persuasive. Only in a later iteration of the law was equality of access across racial lines affirmed as a condition for receipt of capital.[53]

In 1965, the passage and implementation of Medicare and Medicaid brought about sweeping changes with regard to issues of race and access. Since the country was attempting to move toward a one-tier system of care by financially enfranchising assistance across racial lines, there was increased recognition of the value of these new potential patients. One of the most visible signs was within academic medical institutions, which responded by revamping practices within their entities.

Since Medicare required inpatients to be hospitalized in semi-private rooms with four or fewer beds, the terms "ward service," "clinic service," and "teaching service" were abandoned in favor of other terminology, like "university clinical service" or "semi-private service." Similarly, the term "black" was substituted for "Negro."[54] The most significant advances in integration and equal access were achieved by the double impact of the Civil Rights Act of 1964 and the Medicare legislation of 1965.[55] But the issues of access to health care by minorities would continue to occupy a significant role in the health care debate.

A Philosophical and Functional Shift

The passage of Medicare became a license for hospitals to spend.[56] In the period from 1970 to 1975, Medicare fund expenditures more than doubled, outstripping all previous estimates. The influx of these massive amounts of new federal funds began to fundamentally affect the philosophical and operational profile of hospitals in a variety of ways. For-profit hospitals had to demonstrate benevolence. Voluntary and nonprofit hospitals had to demonstrate that they were efficient, and government hospitals had to demonstrate that they were necessary.[57]

At the same time, an earlier prediction made by President Johnson was realized. In a speech on health care in 1965, he noted that more than a third of the nation's hospital beds were obsolete, and that the activation of the Medicare program would place even more pressure on hospitals to respond with new or rehabilitated facilities. In subsequent studies conducted by a variety of entities,[58] the costs of modernizing the oldest hospitals in major American cities was staggering: $1.25 billion in New York City, $255 million in Chicago, and $90 million in Boston. The challenge to fund these extensive modernizations was, in some instances, more than many municipal governments could manage. As the trends moved increasingly away from the notions of mission toward marketplace, public hospitals saw the writing on the wall: despite long traditions of service and excellence, their very survival was at stake.

Conclusions

More than two decades ago, Senator Hubert Humphrey remarked, "It was once said that the moral test of government is how that government treats those in the dawn of life, the children; those who are in the twilight of life, the elderly; and those in the shadows of life— the sick, the needy, and the handicapped."[59] Though there is no doubt that the American health care system is the world's most technologically advanced, this can be cold comfort for those on the fringes of our society, who have fallen through the safety net.

Over the last hundred years, as the country moved toward a higher level of interdependency and complexity, the federal government has played an increasingly significant role in shaping the trends, culture, and direction of society, and the capacity to define public policy and make it work. The development of the modern and postmodern health care system is one of the most compelling examples of the reshaping of an industry and a civility, predicated on significant and definable federal acts.

In less than three decades, three major pieces of federal legislation—Hill-Burton, Medicare, and Medicaid—set the stage for a massive redistribution of health care delivery financing, and fundamentally altered the way Americans think about and receive health care. The interactions of politics and policy served as key factors in legislative outcomes, and directly impacted the conceptualization of health care and its delivery. While the United States maintains its position as the world's temple of scientific advancement, the continuation of longstanding traditions of American benevolence has reconfigured to a new age, and has faded from altruism's earliest conception and expression in a civil society. The complexities of government have added capacity to address health care delivery, in terms of scale and critical mass. But these complexities, when put into practice, have also subtracted from those obligations and societal intents. What remains, however, is a continuing sense of the utility of scientific advancement to address the human condition and the ongoing obligation to grapple successfully with caring for those in need.

Notes

1. See Michael B. Katz, *In the Shadow of the Poorhouse: A Social History of Welfare in America* (New York: Basic Books, 1986), 52-53, 142-149, 150-163, 259-287; *Women, the State and Welfare*, ed. Linda Gordon (Madison: University of Wisconsin Press, 1990); Charles E. Rosenberg, *The Care of Strangers: The Rise of America's Hospital System* (Baltimore: The Johns Hopkins University Press, 1987), 1-68, 97-122, 142-236, 262-352; D. Rosner, *A Once Charitable Enterprise: Hospitals and Health Care in Brooklyn and New York, 1885-1915* (Princeton, NJ: Princeton University Press, 1982), vii, 1-22, 36-80, 94-145, 187-191; Gertrude Himmelfarb, *On Liberty and Liberalism: The Case of John Stuart Mill* (New York: Random House Children's Books, 1974); John Stuart Mill, *On Liberty*, ed. Gertrude Himmelfarb (New York: Penguin Classics, 1976); Huey P. Long, *Every Man a King* (Chicago: Quadrangle Books, 1964); Robert Dallek, *An Unfinished Life: John F. Kennedy, 1917-1963* (Boston: Little, Brown, 2003); Robert Dallek, *Flawed Giant: Lyndon B. Johnson, 1960-1973* (New York: Oxford University Press, 1998), 189-195, 204-209, 293-298, 307-311; Jeffrey Shesol, *Mutual Contempt: Lyndon Johnson, Robert Kennedy, and the Feud that Defined a Decade* (New York: W.W. Norton, 1997), 237, 240; I. Unger and D. Unger, *LBJ: A Life* (New York: John Wiley & Sons, 1999), 362-367; David G. McCullough, *Truman* (New York: Simon & Schuster, 1993).

2. Rosner, 62-93.

3. Morris J. Vogel, "Patrons, Practitioners, and Patients: The Voluntary Hospital in Mid-Victorian Boston," in *Sickness and Health in America: Readings in the History of Medicine and Public Health*, eds. J.W. Leavitt and R.L. Numbers, 3rd ed. (Madison: University of Wisconsin Press, 1997), 324.

4. Rosner, 80.

5. *Financing of Hospital Care in the United States, Volume I: Factors Affecting the Costs of Hospital Care*, ed. John Hayes (New York: Blakiston, 1954), ix-xv. This first volume is one of three volumes that set out the work of the subsequent Commission, and includes *Prepayment and Community* (Volume II) and *Financing Hospital Care for Low-Income Groups* (Volume III). The volumes are located in the collection of the Center for the Study of Nursing History at the University of Pennsylvania.

6. *Financing of Hospital Care in the United States, Volume III: Financing Hospital Care for Non-Wage and Low-Income Groups*, ed. John Hayes (New York: Blakiston, 1954), 97.

7. Rosemary Stevens, *In Sickness and in Wealth: American Hospitals in the Twentieth Century* (New York: Basic Books, 1989), 258-259.

8. Rosemary Stevens, *American Medicine and the Public Interest* (New Haven, CT: Yale University Press, 1976), 271.

9. Paul Starr, *The Social Transformation of American Medicine: The Rise of a Sovereign Profession and the Making of a Vast Industry* (New York: Basic Books, 1982), 310-311.

10. *Financing of Hospital Care in the United States, Volume II: Prepayment and the Community*, ed. John Hayes (New York: Blakiston, 1954), 124.

11. Stevens, *In Sickness and in Wealth*, 208-215; Dallek, *Flawed Giant*, 196.

12. Stevens, *In Sickness and in Wealth*, 209.

13. *Financing Hospital Care in the United States, Volume I: Factors Affecting the Costs of Hospital Care*, xiii.

14. Ibid. See all three volumes for the detailed recommendations made by the commission.

15. McCullough, *Truman*, 469.

16. Ibid., 480.

17. George Bugbee, *Recollections of a Good Life: An Autobiography* (Chicago: American Hospital Association, The Hospital Research and Educational Trust, 1987), 59-96.

18. Stevens, *In Sickness and in Wealth*, 216.

19. Stevens, *American Medicine*, 269.

20. K.M. Ludmerer, *Time to Heal: American Medical Education from the Turn of the Century to the Era of Managed Care* (New York: Oxford University Press, 1999).

21. J. Hollingsworth and E. Hollingsworth, *Controversy about American Hospitals: Funding, Ownership and Performance* (Washington, DC: American Enterprise Institute for Public Policy Research, 1987), 50.

22. J. Weissman, "Uncompensated Hospital Care: Will It Be There If We Need It," *Journal of the American Medical Association* 276 (10, 1996): 823-828.

23. Ibid., 828.

24. Stevens, *In Sickness and in Wealth*, 216-221.

25. Stevens, *American Medicine*, 510.

26. David McBride, *Integrating the City of Medicine: Blacks in Philadelphia Health Care, 1910-1965* (Philadelphia: Temple University Press, 1989), 195-198.

27. Michael Harrington, *The Other America* (New York: Scribner, 1997).

28. Dallek, *An Unfinished Life*, 640.

29. Stevens, *American Medicine*, 438.

30. Dallek, *An Unfinished Life*, 166.

31. For more on Johnson and Robert Kennedy, see Harris Wofford, *Of Kennedys & Kings: Making Sense of the Sixties* (New York: Farrar, Straus & Giroux, 1980), 234-235, and Shesol, *Mutual Contempt*, 237, 240-241.

32. Dallek, *An Unfinished Life*; Diana Nelson Jones, "Appalachia's War: The Poorest of the Poor Struggle Back," *Pittsburgh Post Gazette*, November 26, 2000.

33. Dallek, *An Unfinished Life*, 166.

34. Katz, 265.

35. Dallek, *An Unfinished Life*, 640.

36. Unger and Unger, 291-292.

37. Shesol, 154.

38. Unger and Unger, 291-294.

39. Dallek, *Flawed Giant*, 69.

40. Ibid., 367.

41. Shesol, *Mutual Contempt*; Wofford, *Of Kennedys & Kings*.

42. Shesol, 240-241; Wofford, 234-235.

43. Shesol, 237.

44. Unger and Unger, 363.

45. Shesol, 237.

46. Unger and Unger, 364.

47. Dallek, *Flawed Giant*, 207-208.

48. Unger and Unger, 365.

49. Ibid., 366.

50. Ludmerer, 222-223.

51. See James McPherson's essay, "The Second American Revolution," in *Major Problems in the Civil War and Reconstruction*, ed. Michael Perman (Boston: Houghton Mifflin, 1998) for a description of the post-Civil War legislative actions taken by Southern states to limit the emancipation of black Americans. Also in Perman, for more background see chapters 12-14.

52. Stevens, *In Sickness and in Wealth*, 399, n56.

53. *Congressional Quarterly Almanac*, 1965.

54. Ludmerer, 228-229.

55. Stevens, *In Sickness and in Wealth*, 254.

56. Ibid., 284.

57. Ibid., 285.

58. Stevens, *American Medicine*, 511-512.

59. Hubert Humphrey, in a speech at the dedication of the Hubert Humphrey Building, November 1, 1977, *The Congressional Record*, November 4, 1977, vol. 123, p. 37287.

3

The Closure of PGH in Context: Twentieth-Century Trends in Public Hospitals

Beginning in the 1930's and continuing throughout the next several decades, trends favoring the proliferation of voluntary and proprietary hospitals over public hospitals emerged. The trends were manifested by patients' choice to avoid public hospital care; financing packages that all but prohibited participation by public hospitals; and governance models that, at times, shunned their charitable histories. Philadelphia General Hospital was not the only public hospital threatened by these trends. Several reports as well as specific case examples highlight the implications of the challenges that faced public hospitals throughout the 20th century.

The Emergence of a Trend

The Pennsylvania Hospital and Survey Plan, generated in 1941 by the Commonwealth of Pennsylvania, inventoried the hospitals within the state.[1] The survey, which analyzed hospital data in the Commonwealth back to 1700, revealed a high-water mark of nine government-owned hospitals founded between 1891 and 1900, and a decrease to two founded between 1941 and 1947, for a total aggregate of 49 government-owned hospitals surviving in 1947. This con-

trasts with the founding of nonprofit hospitals, which had a high of
44 in the same decade (1891-1900), for a total aggregate of 209 in
1947. Similarly, proprietary hospitals, which were almost unheard
of (one was founded between 1851 and 1900), began appearing with
increasing frequency in each decade beginning in 1901, and out-
paced government hospital growth in the 1920's, reaching a total of
60 (see Appendix A).[2]

The continuation of this trend was documented in a 1969 report
by the National Forum on Hospital and Health Affairs called *The
Changing Composition of the Hospital System*.[3] The study considered
a variety of hospital influences, including ownership and its implications. Conducted by Duke University, the section on the public hospital system concluded that "There is a need for new thinking regarding public policy, for flexibility, and adaptation to change if public
charity hospitals are to find their proper place in the scale of comprehensive services the public will demand. . . . If they do not meet
these challenges head on, they will not, and should not survive."[4]

In a subsequent and more complex study, Hollingsworth and
Hollingsworth compared the funding, ownership, and performance
of American hospitals (Appendix B) and further illuminated the
movement away from public hospitals.[5] The study extrapolated the
sample size predicated on existing ratios of hospitals by group, and
adjusted for number of beds per hospital. In 1935, the survey recorded an average of 156 beds in public hospitals, 92 in voluntary hospitals, and 23 in proprietary hospitals.[6] In 1961, 5,042 hospital beds
were categorized by 124 in public hospitals, 139 in voluntary hospitals, and 45 in proprietary hospitals,[7] and in 1979 the study recorded 116 in public hospitals, 210 in voluntary hospitals, and 115 in
proprietary hospitals.[8]

In 1976, the Commission on Public-General Hospitals was
established, the same year the closure of PGH was announced. This
commission, an independent body drawn from affiliates of the American Hospital Association and supported by several foundations, had
a twofold mission: to examine the present health care delivery roles
of public general hospitals and to identify their future roles, if any;
and to work toward the generation of a public dialogue that would
enable and encourage policy-makers to address more effectively the
problems and the options for the future of public hospitals. In its
yearlong study, *The Future of the Public-General Hospital: An Agenda*

for Transition, the commission noted that one third of the 5,679 hospitals in operation were public general hospitals.[9] This reflected all hospitals that operated with some component of local, state, or regional government ownership.

The conclusions drawn by the commission were reexamined in a later study conducted by the Alpha Center, a Washington-based health policy group,[10] which validated the value and importance of public hospitals but outlined multiple factors that contributed to the decision to keep or close a public general hospital. The study noted that public hospitals in the 1970's faced oppressive financial burdens that were threatening their survival.[11] The Alpha Center study reviewed several hospitals and health care systems as case studies, including PGH, and identified 15 factors that should be considered when deciding to keep or close a public hospital. The authors broke these factors down into two groups, eight internal factors and seven external factors.

The internal factors included the financial condition of the hospital; the management and administrative problems associated with government bureaucracy; the condition of the physical plant and equipment; the ability to raise capital; the ability to attract adequate and competent staff; the ability to attract patients; the effects of the teaching programs on the operation of the hospital; and the attitude of the board and/or government officials toward the hospital. The external factors included the attitude of the citizenry toward the facility; the fiscal condition of the county or municipality; the attitude of private community clinics; the extent to which the hospital is a source of employment for inner city residents; the overall supply of hospital beds in the community; and the demographic and health status characteristics of the county or municipality. In the case study summary of PGH, each of these factors was addressed, but without great detail and in less detail than the other hospitals selected for the Alpha Center review.

These studies clearly demonstrated a trend away from public hospitals, and toward voluntary and nonprofit hospitals, with proprietary hospitals gaining a smaller measure of critical mass over time. Further, the constructs of the Alpha Center study challenged the prospect for the continued existence of public hospitals. A more in-depth analysis of these factors, as they relate to PGH, bears further consideration.

The Rise of Bureaucracy

In the post-Depression period, hospitals began to move more toward a big-business model, which required a big-business approach.[12] The advent of increased bureaucratization and professionalization via the Civil Service brought to the hospital setting a new, elite leadership class: the professionalized bureaucrat. The profile of these new administrators advanced early notions of benevolence and efficiency to new levels. Their predecessors were often drawn from one of two types: first, the elite and wealthy who offered their services as part of a larger civic obligation; and second, the political bosses who gathered spoils for their constituents.[13] But the new managers were college-educated men of distinction who were encouraged to bring a business orientation to benevolence. Notions of production, profitability, yardsticks, and time and motion studies began to creep into the lexicon of hospital management, signaling another shift in the care of the ill, and by extension, the poor.[14]

Beyond PGH

The 1920 charter change that redistributed PGH populations of the mentally ill to Byberry and the well-poor to Holmesberg[15] signaled a shift in society's view of caring for the poor. The differentiation of illness and wealth was an early indicator of a shifting societal view, a consolidation of focus and power by the discipline of medicine,[16] and the cross-fertilization of the concepts of efficiency and benevolence.[17] The consolidation of power, efficiency, and bureaucracy was repeated in other governmental policy venues, giving rise to a new era of the roles and perceptions of government.[18]

In the early 20th century, the reorientation of hospitals toward a business model hallmarked by notions of efficiency was one of the earliest indicators that hospitals were moving in new directions, and was an early predictor of what would follow. For example, at a contentious board meeting of St. Luke's Hospital in Kansas City in 1917, the leadership adopted a new policy that limited hospital admissions to paying patients who were under the care of the hospital medical staff. The management of the hospital was restructured to include a decision-making body that assigned permission for charity care, prompting the superintendent of nurses to resign.[19]

Charity Hospital, a mission-oriented hospital in New Orleans, is a rather unique case of a privately owned institution that was acquired by the State of Louisiana. It was, and is, one of the few state-owned public hospitals. This may be related to a historic political tradition of commitment to the common man.[20] In the 1980's, when public hospital closures and conversions were happening with increasing regularity across the country, approximately 30 percent of Charity Hospital's patient population was funded by Medicare/Medicaid, and 10 percent were Blue Cross/self-pay patients. The remaining 60 percent was funded by the State of Louisiana. Multiple management efficiencies were introduced at the hospital, but administrators still faced contract rigidity processes and cumbersome purchasing systems.[21] Current budget deficits in the State of Louisiana make this an ongoing point of review.[22]

In a few large cities, freestanding public hospitals became linked into public hospital systems. In 1970, the New York state legislature formed a quasi-independent New York City Health and Hospitals Corporation (HHC). The HHC's 16-member board of directors oversees over 8,000 beds in 12 municipal hospitals, 29 ambulatory care clinics, and four neighborhood-based family health centers.[23] By moving in this direction, the legislature created economies of scale, allowing the HHC as a quasi-governmental agency to develop a $1 billion, ten-year capital plan in 1980, thus permitting consolidation of services and enhanced cohesive capital improvements. While the HHC appeared to do better than many other freestanding public hospitals, there continued to be criticism about mounting deficits, poor quality, and rapid turnover of board and administrative leadership. The political nature of the board is often cited.[24]

By the time Rudolph Giuliani was elected Mayor of New York City in 1995, the HHC was widely disregarded. Poor quality and poor access, mounting deficits, failing physical plant, and political patronage and interference were the characterizations used to describe the public hospital system. These phenomena came on the heels of notions of reinventing government and privatization, embraced in varying degrees in multiple public policy venues. This backdrop set the stage for one of the largest privatizations ever undertaken by a municipal government of its hospitals.[25]

Boston City Hospital (BCH), which in many ways may be the most analogous to Philadelphia General Hospital, was an urban public hospital with more than 1,200 beds in the 1960's, and served as a major teaching institution for three medical schools—Harvard, Tufts, and Boston University. By 1980, BCH had eliminated more than 800 beds and faced a massive deficit of $38 million. The 1981 passage of Proposition $2^1/_2$ eroded the tax base for all public services in the Commonwealth of Massachusetts, resulting in the hospital's losing more than half of its annual subsidy from the City of Boston. Concurrent Medicaid cuts of 20 percent resulted in the recommendation of the Commissioner of Health and Hospitals that BCH be closed to prevent the city from going bankrupt, unless an alternative could be found and implemented. The implementation of a hospital-based HMO, the Boston Health Plan, began in 1981.[26] In 1996, BCH merged with a neighboring university hospital, Boston University Medical Center. The merged institution became Boston Medical Center. Although this new institution confronts contemporary health care delivery dilemmas, a variation of its historic tradition of caring for the poor continues through the use of federal demonstration project funding for the otherwise uninsured and indigent.[27]

Emerging Governance Options for Public Hospitals

Over the last few decades, public hospitals have sought a variety of options to keep their doors open. Restructuring became a key approach to protecting their survival. A new set of models for public hospitals evolved.[28] These are discussed below.

The Traditional Model

Increasingly rare, this is the direct operation of a hospital by a state or local government. The hospital has no independent legal identity. It may exist with or without a separate advisory board. Traditional public hospital models still exist in California, New Mexico, Illinois, and Minnesota.

A Modification of the Traditional Model

This model includes a separate board within a governmental entity that gives the board defined responsibility for the daily operations of the public institution. This permits a higher level of autonomy. These modified models can be found in Massachusetts, Colorado, New York, Michigan, Arizona, and California.

Hospital Authority

The implementation of a hospital authority is another alternative that has been used by some public hospitals. This type of governing authority is often regarded as a quasi-governmental agency and, in many states, requires special legislation to permit its establishment. It becomes, in effect, its own local government with a separate board often appointed by elected officials. Hospital authorities have been created in Tennessee, Georgia, Hawaii, Virginia, Louisiana, Florida, and Colorado.

Hospital District

The creation of a hospital district has been considered as a feasible alternative. A hospital of this model becomes an independent instrumentality of the state, with defined geographic boundaries, taxing authority, and elected board members, similar to some types of school districts. The states of Texas and Florida currently have hospital districts.

Public Benefit Corporations

This is another emerging "boutique" type of entity. These alternatives to traditional nonprofits do not exist in every state and require special enabling legislation. New York City Health and Hospitals Corporation is currently one of the largest public benefit corporations. Several other states have enabling legislation pending.

Nonprofit Corporations

Often, when a public hospital converts to a nonprofit, the conversion is achieved through a contractual agreement with local government and operates under its state's nonprofit corporation statute. Public hospitals in Maryland, Texas, Ohio, Georgia, Michigan, Tennessee, Missouri, and West Virginia have pursued this restructuring option.

Sale, Lease, and/or Management Contract

Under this restructuring plan, public hospitals transfer and/or merge their assets and obligations with an existing entity. Public hospitals in New Mexico, Massachusetts, Michigan, Texas, the District of Columbia, Wisconsin, Kentucky, and Indiana have instituted these types of restructuring in their public hospitals.[29]

The Current Status of Public Hospitals

A recent survey by the National Association of Public Hospitals and Health Systems[30] examined the status of its constituent members from a number of vantage points. The members' principal concern was financial viability and survival. Most of the public hospitals surveyed operated at break-even margins, and that fragile stability had been further eroded by the anticipation of additional cuts in state Medicaid programs, disproportionate share (DSH) payment cuts, and cuts to Medicare Indirect Medical Education (IME) payments that took effect in FY 2003. Other concerns included the inability to negotiate lower pharmaceutical costs; avoidance of new programs that appear to be reforms but are vehicles for the elimination of state/federal partnerships that enhance coverage; the need to expand coverage through Medicaid and CHIP programs, which are important in limiting unreimbursed care for providers of last resort; and the importance of ensuring financing for emergency preparedness so that the fiscal integrity of these public health infrastructures are protected.[31]

The survey, which included 81 public hospitals and health care systems and represented more than 30,000 staffed inpatient beds and more than 8.5 million inpatient days, traced its most recent contact of negative governmental impact to the Balanced Budget Act (BBA). The BBA, a federal law enacted in 1997, required the balancing of the federal budget over five years. This act resulted in significant cuts in Medicare and Medicaid,[32] with the predictable impact on public hospitals evidenced in their continued fiscal instability.

Conclusions

Public hospitals have played a key role in defining our society's altruistic commitment to caring for the least fortunate and were an important venue in which these sentiments found expression in public policy. Shifting societal views, in the past and present, have redefined our public policy approach. As social foundations shift, the institutions built upon them may crumble unless they are reinforced or rebuilt. The story of the closure of PGH lies within the resulting chasm.

Notes

1. Survey Staff of the Pennsylvania Committee on Hospital Facilities, Organization and Standards, *The Pennsylvania Hospital Survey and Plan* (Harrisburg, 1949).

2. Ibid., 6. Since the data for this analysis were collected retrospectively as part of a descriptive research study, it is difficult to assess the adequacy and consistency of the data collection methods.

3. National Forum on Hospital and Health Affairs, *The Changing Composition of the Hospital System* (Durham, NC: Duke University Press, 1969).

4. Ibid., 15.

5. J. Hollingsworth and Ellen Jane Hollingsworth, *Controversy about American Hospitals: Funding, Ownership and Performance* (Washington, DC: American Enterprise Institute for Public Policy Research, 1987), 1-150.

6. Ibid., 90.

7. Ibid., 98.

8. Ibid., 104. The authors of this study note that the statistical significance of their study, reflected in the tables on pages 98 and 104, is 0.001, since the use of aggregate data does not permit tests of significance.

9. Commission on Public-General Hospitals, *The Future of the Public-General Hospital: An Agenda for Transition* (Chicago: Hospital Research and Educational Trust, 1978), 12.

10. M. Isaacs, K. Lichter, and C. Lipschultz, *The Urban Public Hospital: Options for the 1980's* (Bethesda, MD: Alpha Center, 1982), 29-33. The Alpha Center, located in Washington, DC, is a nonprofit health policy center dedicated to improving access to affordable health care.

11. Ibid., ix-x.

12. See Susan Reverby, *Ordered to Care: The Dilemma of American Nursing, 1850-1945* (New York: Cambridge University Press, 1987), 180-207; Rosemary Stevens, *American Medicine and the Public Interest* (New Haven, CT: Yale University Press, 1976).

13. See Harry F. Dowling, *City Hospitals: The Undercare of the Underprivileged* (Cambridge, MA: Harvard University Press, 1982), 16-19, 36-40, 43-44; Michael B. Katz, *In the Shadow of the Poorhouse: A Social History of Welfare in America* (New York: Basic Books, 1986), 157-158.

14. Reverby, 143-149; D. Rosner, "Doing Well or Doing Good: The Ambivalent Focus of Hospital Administration," in *The American General Hospital: Communities and Social Contexts*, eds. Diana E. Long and Janet Golden (Ithaca, NY: Cornell University Press, 1989), 157-169.

15. Ibid.

16. Janet Dieckmann, *Caring for the Chronically Ill: Philadelphia, 1945-1965*, ed. Stuart Bruchey (New York: Garland Publishing, 1999), 47, 52-53, 364; Stevens, *American Medicine and the Public Interest*, 517-519, 34-85; Dowling, 81-83; Katz, 102-113.

17. See Charles E. Rosenberg, *Explaining Epidemics and Other Studies in the History of Medicine* (Cambridge, UK: Cambridge University Press, 1992), 178-215;

Rosenberg, "Social Class and Medical Care in 19th Century America: The Rise and Fall of the Dispensary," in *Sickness and Health in America: Readings in the History of Medicine and Public Health*, eds. Judith Walzer Leavitt and Ronald L. Numbers, 3rd ed. (Madison: University of Wisconsin Press, 1998), 309-322; Katz, 102-113; Rosemary Stevens, *In Sickness and in Wealth: American Hospitals in the Twentieth Century* (New York: Basic Books, 1989), 3-51, 105-366.

18. S. Skowronek, *Building a New American State: The Expansion of National Administrative Capacities, 1877-1920* (New York: Cambridge University Press, 1982), 177-211; P. Baker, "The Domestication of Politics: Women and American Political Society, 1780-1920," in *Women, the State, and Welfare*, ed. L. Gordon (Madison: The University of Wisconsin Press, 1990), 55-91.

19. Joan E. Lynaugh, "From Respectable Domesticity to Medical Efficiency: The Changing Kansas City Hospital, 1875-1920," in *The American General Hospital: Communities and Social Contexts*, eds. D.E. Long and J. Golden (Ithaca, NY: Cornell University Press, 1989), 21.

20. This historical public policy trend, hallmarked by the late Governor Huey Long, who was well known for his massive public works projects, included construction of modern hospitals preceding Hill-Burton. For more information, refer to his autobiography: Huey P. Long, *Every Man a King* (Chicago: Quadrangle Books, 1964).

21. Isaacs, Lichter, and Lipschultz, 75-76.

22. "Belt-Tightening at Charity," *The Times-Picayune*, July 28, 2002, p. 4.

23. Isaacs, Lichter, and Lipschultz, 69-71.

24. Ibid., 71.

25. Maria K. Mitchell, "Privatizing New York City's Public Hospitals: The Politics of Policy Making" (Ph.D. dissertation, The City University of New York, 1998).

26. Isaacs, Lichter, and Lipschultz, 55-57.

27. Randall R. Bovbjerg, Jill A. Marsteller, and Frank C. Ullman, *Health Care for the Poor and Uninsured after a Public Hospital's Closure or Conversion* (Washington, DC: The Urban Institute, September 2000), 10, 13-15.

28. Anne B. Camper, Larry S. Gage, Barbara Eyman, and Steven K. Stranne, *The Safety Net in Transition, Monograph II: Reforming the Legal Structure and Governance of Safety Net Hospitals* (Washington, DC: National Association of Public Hospitals and Health Systems, 1996).

29. Ibid., 33.

30. Ingrid Singer, Lindsay Davison, and Lynne Fagnani, *America's Safety Net Hospitals and Health Systems: Results of the 2001 Annual Member Survey* (Washington, DC: National Association of Public Hospitals and Health Systems, 2003).

31. Ibid., vii.

32. Ibid., 15-17.

4

PGH: Descent and Demise

Near-Death Experiences

This has been the most dismal $1^1/_2$ months I have spent at PGH. . . . psychiatry was a pleasure [and] pulmonary medicine was satisfactory. . . the nursing is fair to good, [but] the attendings were mediocre . . .Special medicine was a joke. . . the nursing is very good, but [the medical supervision] is laughable. . .Female medicine is a disgrace. The residents and attendings are good, and people manage to get fair medical attention, but the nursing care is abominable, and the aides are cruel and sadistic. The intern schedule is criminal. I feel strongly that no one should have to work 56 hours in a row. The patients on this ward [neurology] and the staff. . .who take care of them will people my nightmares for years to come [excerpted from a confidential review by a departing PGH medical resident[1]].

While the history of Philadelphia General Hospital is steeped in scientific discovery, medical advancement, and a commitment to benevolent care, over time these traditions unraveled. Many factors contributed to the descent and demise of the traditions of excellence. As noted in Chapter 2, health care delivery was moving from self-pay to insurance-based "covered lives," causing large-scale changes in delivery and access for most Americans. The advent of Blue Cross as the primary insurer for employer-based coverage laid a broad foundation for more and better coverage for working-class citizens. Unions began to include health care benefits in negotiations with

41

employers. Missing in that equation were the poor and the aged. Multiple small steps toward federal assistance for those less fortunate, beginning with the Lanham Act, were debated in Congress and advanced by Presidents across the span of the early to mid-20th century. Later changes at the federal level contributed mightily to dramatic shifts in financing. The Great Society programs of the 1960's under President Johnson, including Medicare and Medicaid, were the principal drivers of this movement, which presaged the rise of nonprofits and fostered new levels of institutional complexity.[2]

Later a downturn in the national economy during the Nixon administration led to high interest rates, and wage and price controls, which affected the capital markets and put significant pressure on the hospital industry. Urban areas faced record budget deficits and rising demands. The public conversation on the future of American cities was increasingly bleak. New York City edged toward bankruptcy, and the city's public hospitals were identified as one of the most significant drains on its urban economy. At the same time, states were codifying new approaches, such as tax-exempt financing, so hospitals could modernize their high rates of nonconforming beds and expand their access to state-of-the-art technology for diagnostics and treatment.[3]

All of these phenomena produced much roiling within the emerging hospital industry. The severe tumult that ensued was bound to produce casualties. In Philadelphia, PGH—already in a weakened institutional state—became a fatality.

Institutional Complexity

Throughout the late 1960's and early 1970's, the problems associated with managing multi-institutional relationships were apparent. PGH, a city hospital, was dependent on the annual cycle of city funding that was proposed by the administration and passed by City Council. The funding appropriated was the basis for finalizing complex contracts with medical schools, including the University of Pennsylvania, Thomas Jefferson University, and Hahnemann University. Although each of these university-based medical schools had their own hospitals, they contracted with the city to provide care and to serve as a key component in the medical education of interns and residents who rotated into and out of PGH. Often the negotiations of these contracts would stall for months. Portions of agreements would not be honored. Discrepancies emerged over payments and schedules. Tensions among the schools presented themselves in negotiations over which institutions would handle what services, and which services would have equipment purchases made in increasingly tight budget cycles. There were also tensions and unresolved issues regarding the allocation of the new funding streams associated with Medicare and Medicaid.

The negotiations surrounding these contracts were often so protracted that one contract cycle would end, and another ensue, before completion of the preceding year's contract. In 1968, David Maxey, an attorney representing the University of Pennsylvania (PENN) in its contract negotiations, sought to persuade the assistant city solicitor that an 18-month contract would be preferable. But the Solicitor, Isador Kranzel, asserted that the city did not have the power to adopt more than a 12-month contract without passage of an ordinance by City Council.[4] Correspondence from that year documented the ongoing debates related to contract amounts and methods for seeking an adjustment via the Ad Hoc Committee for additional compensation.[5]

In the larger world, the sense that PGH was not on firm footing was also brought to bear in these negotiations. In a letter to Alfred Beers, the business manager at the University of Pennsylvania, attorney Maxey wrote: "As far as I can tell, the 1969-70 contract with the City has not moved at all in the past three months. There are newspaper reports, as you certainly know, to the effect that the City would like to turn over the PGH—lock, stock, and barrel—to some private institution. Those reports are sufficient indication to me that the City is not prepared to give adequate funding to the operation of the PGH for the next fiscal year. . . I continue to recommend that we keep the pressure up, so that if and when negotiations begin, the City will have a hard time claiming that the University has not made its position entirely clear."[6]

At the same time, the University of Pennsylvania was seeking to cope internally with its ongoing cash flow problems. In a letter dated March 27, 1969, Alfred Beers wrote to comptroller Charles Farrell: "I am writing to you at Dean Gelhorn's request. . . you are correct in that this budget could be underfunded by $19,446. Whether or not a deficit occurs, will not be known until after June 30, 1969, when the expenditures for all three medical schools involved in patient care activities in PGH are compared with the expenditure ceiling imposed on us by the City of Philadelphia . . . I do not believe any surplus will exist, because of the arbitrary manner in which the expenditure ceiling was conceived by the office of the Health Commissioner, and PENN will probably be required to absorb this deficit, which is becoming somewhat of a habit for us. . . . Since negotiations for a one-year contract with the City will be entered into shortly, it is imperative that someone take a long hard look at the City's proposition so that we can perhaps cease our subsidizing of a City-owned hospital, which I don't think we can afford to do."[7]

Farrell responded to Beers on March 28, writing: "The agreement of the School of Medicine to fund the potential overdraft in the PGH operating account will allow us to process the PGH operating budget for the six month period, ending June 30, 1969. Should the School of Medicine continue to agree to fund overdrafts in the PGH Operating Account, it could conceivably arrive at the point where the surplus funds would be exhausted. It seems appropriate to me that the PGH funding problem should be resolved at the earliest possible date. . . ."[8]

There were other problems on the contract horizon. In a letter to Dean Gelhorn at the University of Pennsylvania Medical School dated January 21, 1969, David Maxey advised the dean of the city's intention to change its contracting procedures. According to Isador Kranzel, Maxey advised the dean that all three institutions—PENN, Jefferson, and Hahnemann—would operate on the basis of one contract, as opposed to three separate contracts, as was the prevailing practice. "Moreover," Maxey added, "to the extent the adjustments need to be made throughout the year depending on the needs of the three institutions involved, and the amount of work which each one has undertaken, it will be more difficult, in my judgment, to effect a satisfactory settlement if we are working in the context of a one contract document."[9]

In June 1969, 13 days before the end of the fiscal year, the contracts between PENN and PGH were still not signed. Maxey received a message from Kranzel's office that he could not send out contracts for execution, since the staffing patterns must be attached to the contract, and there was not yet agreement between PGH and PENN on staffing. He also informed Maxey through his secretary that he had no authority to address balances owed to PENN from 1967 and 1968.

On June 23, 1969, Alfred Beers sent correspondence to Edward Martin, Director of Finance for the City of Philadelphia, and to Ernest Zeger, Administrative Services Director for PGH. In these letters, Beers asserted that he was sending two invoices from the University of Pennsylvania for contract years 1967 and 1968, totaling almost $65,000 for patient care services performed by the PENN Division.[10] In a separate letter to David Maxey outlining his correspondence with Martin and Zeger, Beers pointed out to Maxey by his enclosure of minutes, that the Ad Hoc Committee, which is the venue to resolve interinstitutional issues, had agreed to a redistribution of funds across institutional lines, as long as such totals did not exceed the $1.7 million allocation. In this, Beers asserted ". . . savings from the Hahnemann and Jefferson budgets can be applied to the PENN overexpenditure simply by amending the agreement. The preliminary figures contained in the minutes would indicate that Hahnemann and Jefferson probably would have underexpended by a sufficient amount to cover the PENN overexpenditure."[11]

Over the next several months there was continuing correspondence reflecting disagreements over the amounts of reimbursement due the University.[12] These disagreements found expression in other significant interagency venues.[13] The PGH Budget Committee, the Ad Hoc Committee, and the Long-Range Planning Committee became forums for unresolved management issues. In a 1969 letter to executive director Elton Barclay, Dr. Harvey Brodovsky voiced his ongoing frustration with the decision-making and limited capacity of the Budget Committee to act, saying: "It was apparent that the chairmen of the PGH departments did not know what their budget was for the year 1969-70. It seems incomprehensible to us that any department head should be expected to function in this manner. Would you therefore instruct your staff to provide these department heads with a copy of the specific budget for their department, and to explain these budgets if necessary. . . A year ago the Medical Staff adopted a set of rules outlining the composition and the function of the budget committee. . . A copy of this is enclosed. It is our feeling that these rules should be adopted by hospital administration and that the budget committee of the medical staff should function as outlined in the enclosed set of rules."[14]

In addition to interagency financial disagreements, there were also differences about devising new architecture to try to manage distribution of new federal resources. In 1967, the city sought an agreement with the medical schools to establish one fund, the Professional Services Fund Account, which would receive reimbursement from Medicare Part B payments associated with physician services provided at PGH.[15] Over a two-year period, meetings were held that resulted in complex financial formulas and layers of administrative and bureaucratic decision-making.[16] The eventual plan was that the Budget Committee, in consultation with the Ad Hoc Committee and each of the departments, would allocate the funds toward programmatic needs, including supplies, equipment, and a variety of related services. The departments were expected to prioritize and communicate those priorities, which would necessarily compete with not only other departments, but also other institutions. There was continuing disagreement about how or even whether this could be accomplished. In a letter dated February 12, 1969, two years from the date of the first draft, Dr. Malcolm Cates wrote to Elton Barclay that "From my conversations with other physicians, it is my understanding the Internal Revenue Service will hold the physician responsible for such fees, even though they are turned over to the parent institution. I have discussed this with my accountant, who has urged that I defer joining this plan until all aspects of it have been fully developed."[17] Two days later, Dr. Brodovsky from Jefferson Medical College also wrote to Barclay, stating, "I believe it would be unwise to sign this [the Professional Services Fund form] until we have received a favorable ruling from the Internal Revenue Service, and until the collections department shows how it intends to bill, where the doctor's name will appear, etc."[18]

The lines of conflict across institutions, revolving around the financial benefits to which they hoped to lay claim, were drawn. The difficulty with which PGH, the city, and the participating medical schools attempted to navigate these new funding streams emanating from Johnson's Great Society programs was, in many ways, a harbinger of things to come.

The Politics of Planning

In 1971, at a meeting of departmental staff in the Department of Medicine, Dr. Truman Schnabel advised those in attendance about an important reversal of fortune for PGH. A proposed $25 million bond issue would not be on the November ballot. The bond issue, scheduled to include a $900,000 planning grant for PGH, was now a casualty.[19] This was significant for a variety of reasons.

First, it was well known that Mayor James Tate was quietly seeking another approach to the management of PGH. In March 1969, he contacted Luther Terry, the vice-president for medical affairs at the University of Pennsylvania, as well as other university officials, to ask if PENN would take over responsibility for the hospital.[20] Both the University and the PGH leadership acknowledged that "something had to be done," and that the hospital was in "great need" of renovations, estimated to cost between $70 million and $100 million.[21] Terry stated that the university would form a committee to examine the issue. While Terry would not speak publicly about the amount of the existing contract with PGH, he was clear in saying that the university would have to evaluate the benefits of such an arrangement. He did not, at that time, allude to the fact that the university had already become the short-term loan agent for operating capital, since PGH had yet to reimburse PENN that year under the existing contract.[22]

Second, the significance of the $25 million bond issue delay went beyond the $900,000 for the PGH planning grant. There were massive changes occurring that realigned the nature of health care delivery in very fundamental ways. As Medicare and Medicaid were implemented, the redirection of now–reimbursable patients toward voluntary/nonprofit beds became an important funding avenue. To achieve that, large-scale capital programs that encompassed updating both the beds and the technology were essential to hospitals' expansion strategies.

Like the nonprofit hospitals that needed updating, PGH was in desperate need of refurbishment, massive physical plant improvements, and new equipment.[23] The costs of capital financing were prohibitive, and philanthropic financing, though an important component, was not enough. The passage of Medicare, which included a small capital allocation for each patient, permitted hospitals to begin to build their internal reserves. But in Philadelphia, one of the most important developments for the city's hospitals came when a new agency with broad financing powers was created: the Hospitals Authority of Philadelphia.

Expansion of the Health Care System and the Rise of Nonprofits

Before 1974, when a Philadelphia nonprofit hospital needed to finance a capital project, it had limited choices. It could try to raise philanthropic dollars; it could accept conventional financing at high interest rates; or it could seek financing from one of a few authorities outside the city with access to tax-exempt financing. Because of the newness of these hybrid entities, municipalities and counties who could enact enabling legislation to create access to tax-exempt capital markets were, understandably, reluctant to provide such financing. That said, the first tax-exempt hospital bond was floated by the Montgomery County Hospital Authority in 1971. Later, in 1973, Frankford Hospital's strategic plan called for the construction of a new patient care wing. Both the Allegheny County Hospital Authority and the Bucks County Hospital Authority declined to issue the bond. The executive director of Frankford Hospital, John Neff, and the hospital's general counsel, John Quinn, had to seek other means to achieve their financing objective. Quinn and Neff, in cooperation with the City Solicitor's Office and with assistance from the Montgomery County Hospital Authority, drafted legislative language. The question of a Philadelphia Authority was now squarely on the agenda.[24]

On September 5, 1973, Philadelphia City Council held public hearings on Mayor Frank Rizzo's proposal to create such an authority for the city's hospitals, making Philadelphia the nineteenth county or municipality to do so. The hearings took testimony from Wharton Shober, the president and CEO of Hahnemann Medical School and Hospital, who reported that 75 percent of Hahnemann's beds were deemed nonconforming.[25] Peter Herbut, president of Thomas Jefferson University, testified that 75 percent of Jefferson's beds were also obsolete, and the rest were deemed non-conforming.[26] He further testified that Jefferson had no other recourse, save creation of the proposed authority, to get access to tax-exempt financing.

Four months later, on January 16, 1974, City Council introduced Bill 1102: "An ordinance authorizing the City of Philadelphia to organize an authority to be known as the Hospitals Authority of Philadelphia, pursuant to the provisions of the Municipal Authorities Act of 1945, P.L. 382, as amended, under certain terms and conditions."[27] Testifying again in favor of the bill were Shober and Herbut, joined this time by John Neff for Frankford Hospital. All represented hospitals that needed immediate financing. Also testifying were University of Pennsylvania vice-president John Heatherston, Joseph Williamson from the Delaware Valley Hospital Association, and many other distinguished members of the Philadelphia business and civic community. Their very presence provided "calculated influence."[28]

An important area of focus in these hearings was the increasing number of empty hospital beds in Philadelphia. Councilman Isidore Bellis questioned Joseph Williamson, president of the Delaware Valley Hospital Council. Williamson, a former hospital administrator and former hospital commissioner for the Commonwealth of Pennsylvania, assured Bellis that safeguards were built into the overbedding issue, since the Hospital Survey Committee had approved only 52 percent of the projects submitted to them. He continued to emphasize the urgency to access needed capital, and stressed that the costs for much-needed modernization were escalating, in part due to inflation, and that the more time passed, the more the necessary capital improvements would cost.[29]

Another significant area of concern, especially to the city administration, was Philadelphia's bond rating.[30] Under Pennsylvania law, the authority had standing as a separate government (or a quasi-governmental) agency. Because of this unique standing, it could offer tax-exempt financing to nonprofit hospitals that would not affect the city's bond rating. Wharton Shober made a point of emphasizing this in his testimony, saying that the use of authority-based financing of a new building for Hahnemann "will not involve the City's credit in any way."[31] The bond rating was important for many reasons. As a general principle, a city's bond rating directly affects the city's ability to borrow money for both short- and long-term financing. The capacity to borrow money is essential to the operation of any municipal government. A favorable bond rating permits the City to borrow at lower rates, thus decreasing the costs of borrowing, and having a direct impact on the cost of doing the business of the municipality. Further, New York City, which was in dire straits financially, was very much on the minds of those involved in the decisions regarding hospital financing. The large, publicly funded municipal hospital system was regarded by many as one of the principal drivers of the fiscal demise of New York City.[32] Shober also challenged the City Council to consider the historic role that Philadelphia has occupied in science and medicine, concluding that ". . . Philadelphia will suffer a major deterioration in its present position of world leadership in medicine" should there be further delay in passage and implementation of an authority.[33]

Council President George Schwartz concluded the hearing, and 55 minutes from the start, the committee on rules adjourned. The bill was reported out of committee the following day and passed without dissent on January 24, 1974. Mayor Rizzo signed it into law on January 28, 1974. The City of Philadelphia would have its own hospitals authority. The fiscal floodgate was swinging open.[34]

During the start-up phase, unanticipated challenges arose. The new authority took over a year to build its systems and develop the working relationships necessary to operate. Despite this, the pent-up demand was clear. By the end of the first year, 12 institutions had applied, or indicated that they would apply, for tax-exempt financing. On September 11, 1975, the Hospitals Authority sold a $34 million issue to assist in the financing of the Silverstein Pavilion at the Hospital of the University of Pennsylvania, scheduled to be a 14-floor ambulatory and inpatient facility. On November 3, the authority issued an $81.6 million bond, the largest in the nation's history of tax-exempt financing, to Thomas Jefferson University Hospital.[35] The following year, on August 1, 1976, the authority issued a $39.5 million bond for Hahnemann's capital program, which included new construction and equipping of a hospital tower, as well as the renovation of existing hospital facilities and refinancing of its debt obligation.[36]

The significance of the modernization and expansion programs of PENN, Jefferson, and Hahnemann could not, or should not, have been lost on PGH executives. The hospitals were all contract partners with PGH to provide medical care and were now invested in a new venture: filling their modernized and technologically superior beds with paying or covered patients. Since the advent of Medicare and Medicaid, that prospect was within reach.

A Convergence of Phenomena and Circumstance

In the early 1970's, the federal and local legislation bore the fruit of their intent: the ubiquitous construction of new, modern community hospitals that were technologically advanced and run by able, college-educated administrators;[37] expansion and development of nonprofit/voluntary teaching hospitals connected with medical schools;[38] massive federal increases in direct funding for the care of the aged, and substantial increases of state/federal funding for the poor;[39] decreases in direct federal aid to cities;[40] decreases in middle-class urban population with the development of the suburbs related to

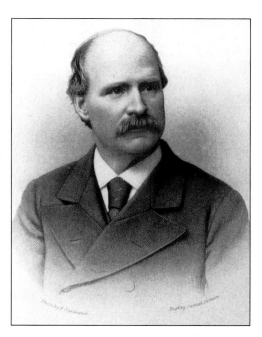

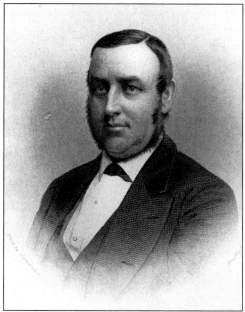

Anthony Drexel (*top*) and George Childs were benefactors of the Philadelphia General Hospital, and were responsible for a wave of early reform, recruiting Florence Nightingale protégé Alice Fisher to PGH to professionalize the delivery of nursing care.
Photos courtesy of the Center for the Study of Nursing History, The University of Pennsylvania

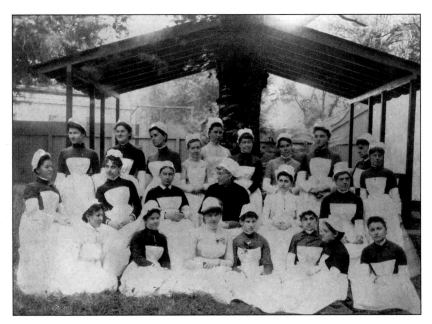

Alice Fisher (*seated, center of middle row, facing left of photo*) with the first graduating class of nurse probationers. *Photo courtesy of the Center for the Study of Nursing History, The University of Pennsylvania*

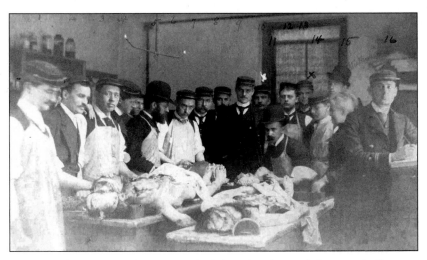

Dr. William Osler, regarded by many as the father of modern pathology, conducting autopsies with medical students in the Green Room at the Philadelphia General Hospital. *Photo courtesy of the Center for the Study of Nursing History, The University of Pennsylvania*

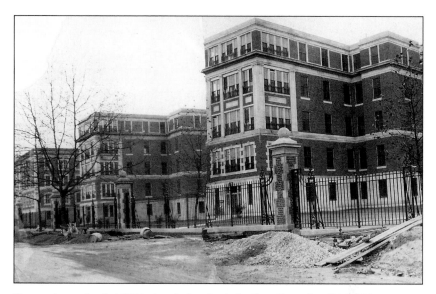

The newly constructed PGH, days before its dedication, November 27, 1927. *Reprinted with permission, The Philadelphia Inquirer*

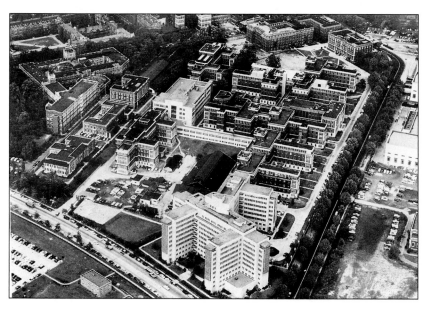

Aerial view, the Philadelphia General Hospital, covering several city blocks. *Reprinted with permission, The Philadelphia Daily News*

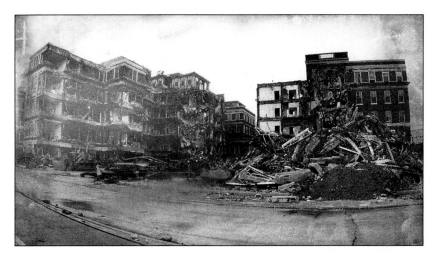

Demolition of the PGH underway, May 29, 1979. *Reprinted with permission*, The Philadelphia Daily News

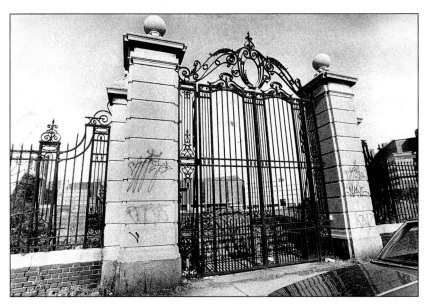

Vacant site still enclosed by the brick and wrought-iron gates, now covered in graffiti, February 12, 1982. *Reprinted with permission*, The Philadelphia Daily News *and* The Philadelphia Inquirer

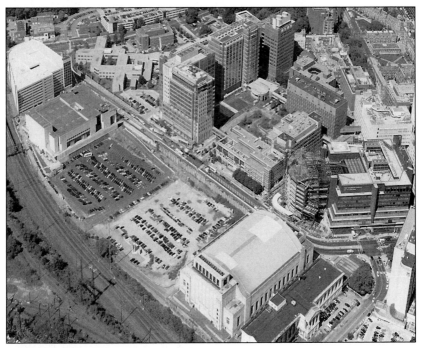

The new Jerusalem: the former PGH site is now occupied by the Children's Hospital of Philadelphia Wood Center; the Madalyn and Leonard Abramson Research Center; the University of Pennsylvania School of Nursing; the Consortium, a mental health facility. Several other research and clinical care buildings also occupy the former PGH site, and more development for a state-of-the-art cancer diagnosis and treatment center is underway. *Photo courtesy of the Children's Hospital of Philadelphia*

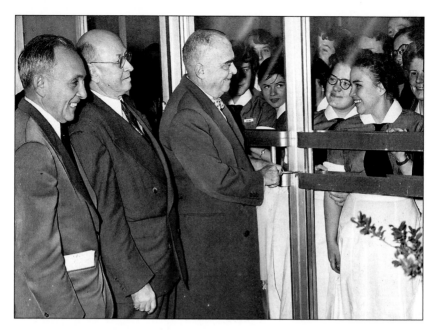

Mayor Bernard Samuel (*center*) and other officials prepare to enter for the dedication of the new $8.5 million neurological building, greeted by student nurses, October 31, 1951. *Reprinted with permission*, The Philadelphia Inquirer

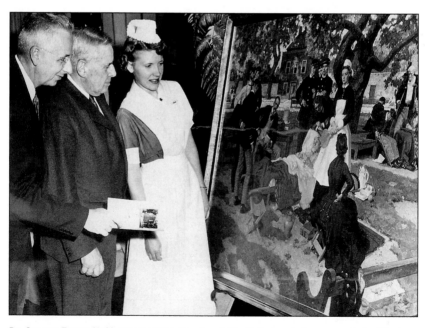

Dr. George Farrar (*left*), the medical director of Wyeth Laboratories presents to Alfred Scattergood, the president of the PGH board of trustees, and student nurse Margaret Delp, the famous "Osler at Old Blockley" painting, June 1953. *Reprinted with permission*, The Philadelphia Inquirer

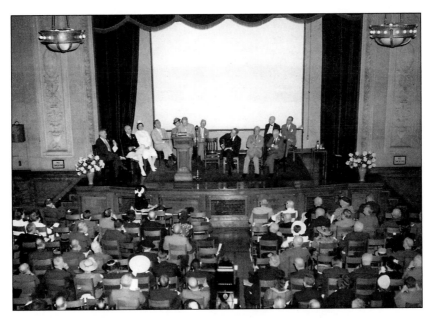

Dr. Joseph McFarland speaks at the dedication of the Osler Memorial Building at the PGH. The Osler Memorial Building served as a historical repository for original Osler memorabilia, much of which is now housed at the College of Physicians, June 1940. *Reprinted with permission,* The Philadelphia Daily News *and* The Philadelphia Inquirer

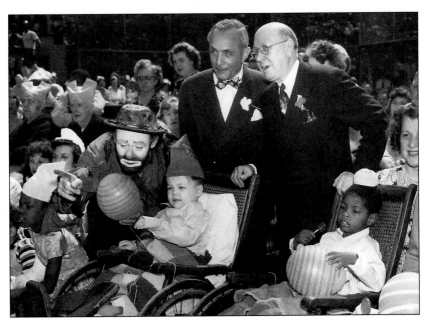

The annual PGH circus was a welcome distraction for the sick children. Here the famous clown Emmett Kelly entertains two of the PGH patients, with Dr. Pasquale Luchessi (*left*) and Rufus Reeves looking on, undated photo. *Reprinted with permission,* The Philadelphia Daily News *and* The Philadelphia Inquirer

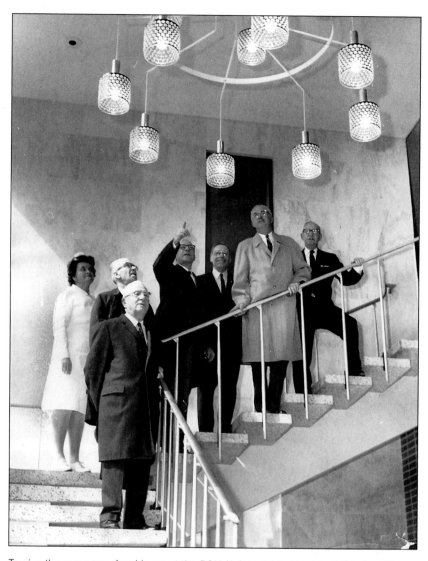

Touring the new nurses' residence at the PGH (*left to right*), Director of Nursing Rita Fenwick; Commissioner of Public Property, Charles Day; architect, Israel Demchick; Managing Director Fred Corleto; Health Commissioner Dr. Norman Ingram; Mayor James Tate; PGH executive director Henry Kolbe (*in foreground*), March 23, 1966.
Reprinted with permission, The Philadelphia Inquirer

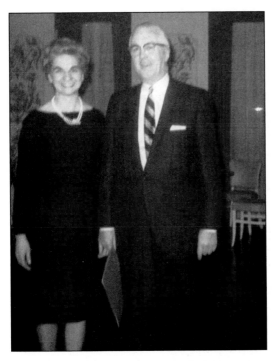

PGH nurses receive a commendation from Mayor James Tate, pictured with Director of Nursing Stephanie Stachniewicz. *Photo courtesy of the Center for the Study of Nursing History, The University of Pennsylvania*

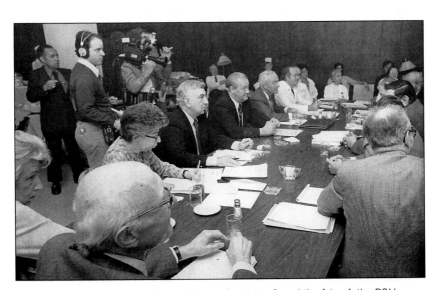

One of the many public meetings to discuss the state of, and the fate of, the PGH. Pictured from the bottom (*left to right*): Earl Perloff, chairman of the board of trustees; Deputy Managing Director Tina Weintraub; unknown woman; John Facenda; Charles Gallagher; John Mullaney; Dr. Heaton; Dr. Storey (*partially obscured behind Dr. Heaton*), February 17, 1976. *Reprinted with permission*, The Philadelphia Daily News

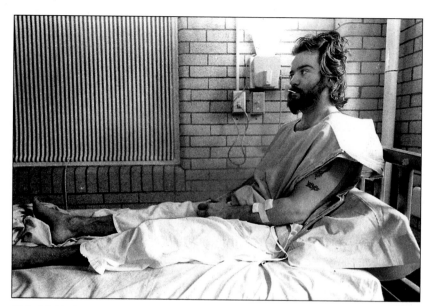

Philadelphia Daily News reporter Hoag Levins on a stretcher, posing as a derelict patient at PGH, as he develops material for the PGH expose, which would reshape the debate about the survival of the institution, January 19, 1986. *Reprinted with permission*, The Philadelphia Daily News

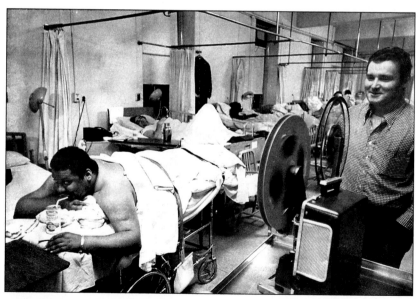

The overcrowded Police and Fireman's Ward during "Movie and Pizza Night." Patients from other units were invited to join recovering police and firefighters for some entertainment, which was sponsored by the Fraternal Order of Police. *Reprinted with permission*, The Philadelphia Daily News and The Philadelphia Inquirer

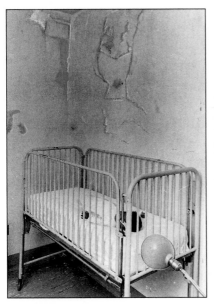

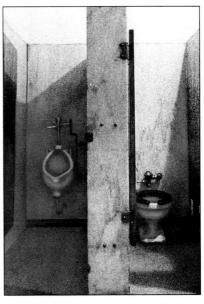

The hospital's physical decline is apparent in the nursery, with cracked and peeling paint over infant cribs...

a "his and hers" bathroom, used by up to forty patients...

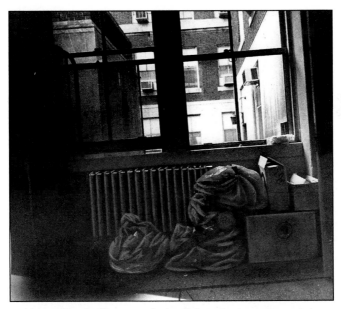

and bags of trash piled up against radiators. *Reprinted with permission,* The Philadelphia Daily News *and* The Philadelphia Inquirer

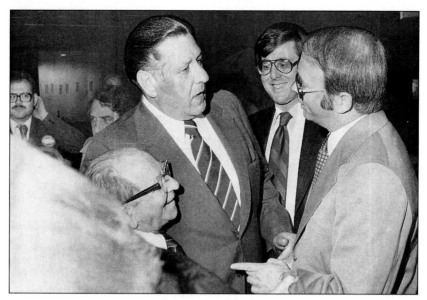

Mayor Frank Rizzo (*top left*) with City Solicitor Martin "Marty" Weinberg (*center*), talking with District Attorney F. Emmet Fitzpatrick. Weinberg was Rizzo's principal political advisor, and counseled against the PGH closure because of political fallout.
Reprinted with permission, The Philadelphia Inquirer

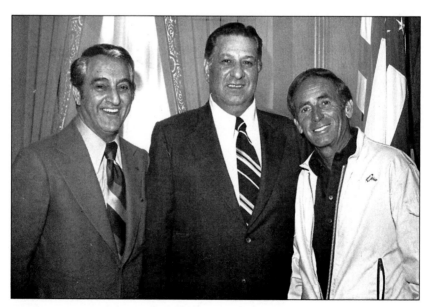

Mayor Rizzo (*center*) with entertainers Danny Thomas (*left*) and Joey Bishop. When celebrities were in town, Rizzo frequently prevailed upon them to visit injured police and firemen at PGH. *Reprinted with permission*, The Philadelphia Daily News *and* The Philadelphia Inquirer

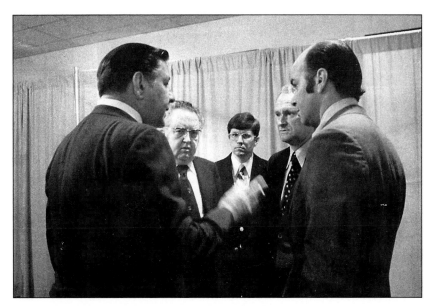

Mayor Rizzo (*left*) with Finance Director Leonard Moak (*standing next to Rizzo*), and Managing Director Hillel "Hilly" Levinson (*in foreground*). Levinson made the announcement of the PGH closure, and was burned in effigy in the ensuing protests. May 1976. *Reprinted with permission*, The Philadelphia Inquirer

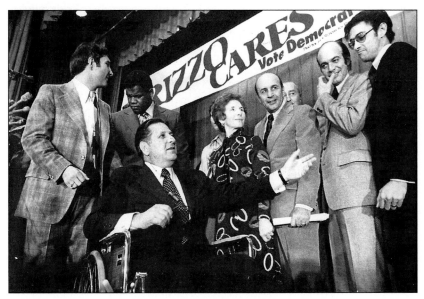

Mayor Rizzo announcing his campaign for reelection: (*left to right*) Frank Rizzo Jr.; Tony Fulwood, the first African American to be assigned to the elite Mayor's Security Unit; Mayor Rizzo (*in wheelchair*), recovering from a broken hip; Carmela Rizzo, wife of the Mayor; State Senator Anthony "Buddy" Cianfranni; Hillel "Hilly" Levinson. *Reprinted with permission*, The Philadelphia Inquirer

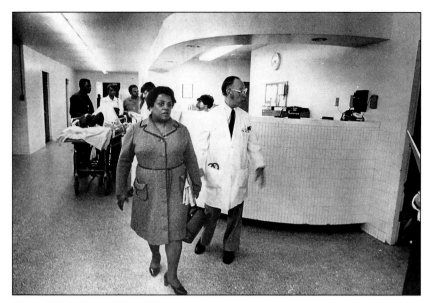

Republican City Councilwoman Dr. Ethel Allen tours the PGH during the period of tumult that preceded the closure. *Reprinted with permission*, The Philadelphia Daily News *and* The Philadelphia Inquirer

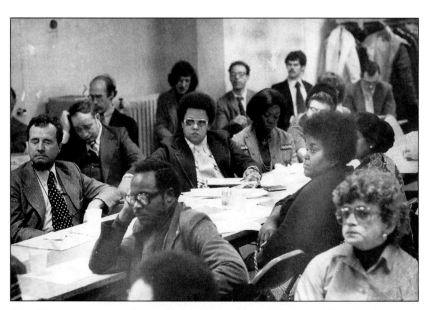

One of the many community meetings to discuss the implications of the closure announcement. *Reprinted with permission*, The Philadelphia Daily News

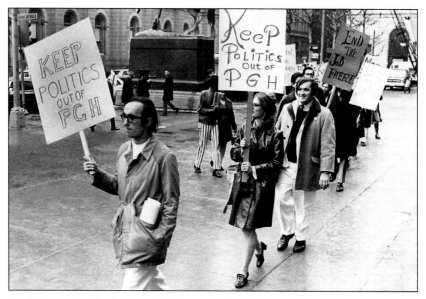

Physicians protest inadequate facilities and seek more patient care support for PGH.
Reprinted with permission, The Philadelphia Daily News

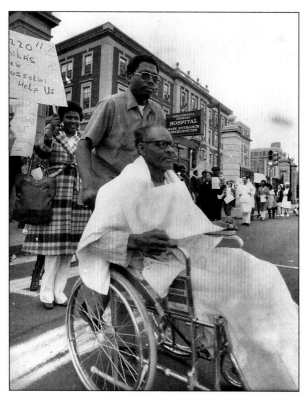

An AFSCME and District Council 33 organized protest at PGH, February 1976.
Reprinted with permission, The Philadelphia Daily News *and* The Philadelphia Inquirer

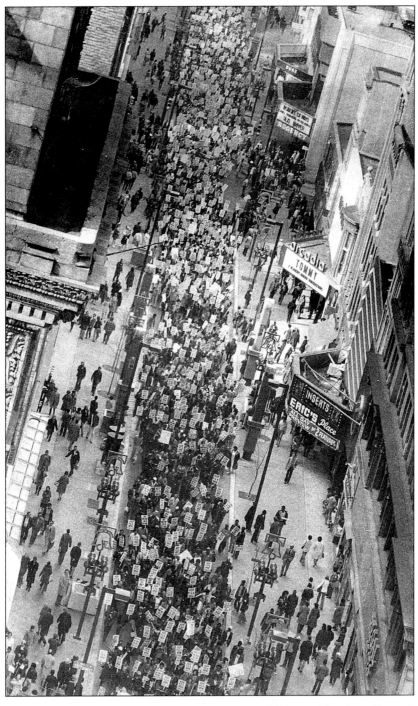

A massive protest rally against the closure, beginning at PGH, marching down Chestnut Street, and culminating at City Hall, February 1976. *Reprinted with permission*, The Philadelphia Inquirer increases in federal road construction and mortgage policies;[41] and aging city structures and fossilized bureaucracies. This was the primordial soup that gave birth to the new health care system, and set the stage for the demise of the Philadelphia General Hospital.

The modernization of hospitals would not have been possible without revenue generated through federal funding mechanisms, which distributed much-needed dollars into the Philadelphia health care industry and, subsequently, redistributed patients. Prior to 1966, health care in the United States was delivered through a two-tiered system.[42] Following 1966, the definition of "patients who could afford the cost of medical care" changed dramatically. Paying patients now were not only those who were more fortunate, but also those who were too poor to afford care. The impoverished and the elderly, along with the more affluent population, were now able to exercise a right to choose a location for hospital care.[43] Patients with less lucrative chronic conditions and those who were substance-addicted continued to be remanded to public hospitals.[44] "Clearly the last resort utilization of the charity hospital was shrinking."[45]

But funding mechanisms, while serving as a catalyst to change, are not the reason that Philadelphia General Hospital closed.[46] After all, the increase in paying patients, theoretically, could have supported growth at PGH as it did at its nonprofit sister institutions.[47] To understand why PGH closed, one must look beyond the financing systems of the time to consequential government actions and societal trends.

Governmental Influences

The history of PGH, as with its other public hospital cohorts, was marked by political influences.[48] Former New York Mayor Ed Koch described the difficulties he faced as he worked to reform his city's public hospital system and the significant political disincentives working against a rational model of allocation of fiscal resources.[49] Public hospitals throughout the nation had histories of mismanagement, political influence, and corruption.[50] During the period following World War II, Philadelphians grew intolerant of political malfeasance.[51] The public demanded reform in general and in health care delivery in particular.[52]

In 1951, Philadelphia voters adopted the Home Rule Charter. Among other requirements, it obligated the city to concern "itself with the health needs of all its people."[53] The charter placed PGH under the auspices of the Department of Public Health. Using ambiguous language, the charter simultaneously divided responsibility between the Philadelphia Board of Health and the PGH Board of Trustees.[54] These ambiguities in leadership would not be clarified throughout the balance of the hospital's existence[55] and contributed mightily to the long-term difficulties of ensuring able institutional management and control.

Given the number of sequential studies, commissions, and panels,[56] one might reasonably assume that it was a mayoral obligation to conduct an overall review. In the two decades preceding the closure, each mayor undertook some form of study or review that made recommendations to reform PGH and health care delivery in Philadelphia. "Often begun in the midst of a controversy about conditions at PGH, the studies slowly proceeded to their conclusions, were eventually published and then promptly forgotten—until the next controversy."[57] In February 1970, Mayor Tate issued a report on municipal hospital services that recapped the findings of the reports of previous administrations. The Hubbard Report, issued by Dr. John Hubbard in 1952 on behalf of the Board of Health, made three key recommendations, including the need for more district health centers to serve as a vital part of the community whose needs they would serve; health maintenance of the family as a unit; and rationalization of national and local financing of care so that there was no "bargain basement care for the indigent. . . while a better quality of care is reserved for the well-to-do."[58]

During the administration of Mayor Joseph Clark, his advisors observed that PGH was still problematic, and urged the mayor to more closely affiliate the running of the hospital with the city's five medical schools. This provoked a firestorm of controversy regarding the preference of the PGH physicians to keep the hospital "independent." The proposal to contract out services lay dormant for five years until the next mayor, Richardson Dilworth, revived the concept. Soon after, the contracts for services were signed.[59] In 1954 under Health Commissioner James Payson Dixon, Vincent Kling was commissioned to evaluate the Northern Division, which was a large, underutilized institution and parcel in North Philadelphia. The subsequent study, the Kling Report of 1955, recommended that the Northern Division be converted into a tuberculosis hospital. The report also noted that caring for the chronically ill was "a staggering problem" because 65,000 citizens were stricken each month by disease. The report also warned of the potential for city overbedding since there had been a 12 percent drop in inpatient care at both branches of PGH from 1931 to 1954.[60]

Mayor Dilworth appointed a blue-ribbon panel led by attorney Morris Duane. The Duane Report, issued in 1957, was described as "a watershed in the development of the City's public policy."[61] The policy committee made two recommendations, both of which were heeded within a year of its issue: first, the final resolution of the medical schools as contractors to deliver care at PGH, with two of the schools dropping out and the remaining three signing contracts; and second, the closing of the Northern Division. This report also opened the door to free or low-cost care, stating, "Promotion of public health is the duty of every civilized community."[62]

One of the most important recommendations in the Duane Report was the subsuming of PGH into the Department of Public Health. The organizational plan stated that the program for medical care of the needy would be under the direction of the Health Commissioner and the day-to-day responsibility for the hospital would be under the direction of the Board of Trustees and the director.[63] While ultimately ill advised, this was a sincere attempt to coordinate and consolidate the needs of the citizens with the resources of the city. Philadelphia moved forward on ambulatory care expansion with some success. But acute care and the contracts with the medical schools to render services at PGH remained a source of consternation and contention. In 1964, the mayor appointed yet another advisory committee, under the leadership of Paul Lefton. The committee's goal was to " try to make. . . contract negotiations with the hospitals coherent."[64] The tug-of-war between the city's resources and the hospital's needs and preferences was apparent. The tensions would continue as each side asserted its position. What neither side may have realized was that these issues would change shape significantly, and soon.

Between 1960 and 1966, the number of beds in use at PGH for acute care dropped and the number of beds committed to long-term care more than doubled.[65] In part, this exodus of acute care was due to physicians contracted by the medical schools to provide care at PGH referring patients to their own school's hospitals, but it was also related to the dissatisfaction with care received at PGH.[66] The resources of Medicare and Pennsycare, Pennsylvania's Medicaid program, allowed less fortunate citizens the opportunity to express their dissatisfaction with the care delivered at PGH[67] by going elsewhere. Hospital usage representing a measurable barometer of satisfaction revealed that "Increasing numbers chose newer and better equipped hospitals."[68] The massive capital rehabilitation that was to be constituted under the aegis of the Philadelphia Hospital Authority, with PGH's major medical school partners, gave choices to Philadelphia patients. And these Philadelphians, without the opportunity at the polls, were voting with their feet.

Based in part on this observation, the 1970 Tate report concluded, "Clearly, the last resort utilization of the charity hospital was shrinking."[69] This led the Hospital Survey Committee in 1967 to pose the question: "Should [PGH] be rebuilt to meet modern standards, or should it be phased out, and other institutions throughout Philadelphia increased in size to provide the services now provided by PGH?"[70]

Medicare, Medicaid, and the Promise Unfulfilled

There was great optimism on a variety of fronts regarding the positive impact that the implementation of Medicare and Medicaid would have on the payment for health care services. But it soon became clear that, though welcome, these reimbursements would not be the much-hoped-for panacea. "By 1968, Medicare was covering 25 percent of PGH hospital patients. Medicaid was providing only $4 per outpatient visit, even though the actual costs were estimated by the hospitals to be closer to $13 per visit."[71] PGH was seeking an additional $8 million to cover unreimbursed costs in addition to the other costs associated with care delivery, including the medical school contracts. Then, in 1969, the Commonwealth declared a fiscal crisis and by executive order increased eligibility standards. Ten of the hospitals under contract with the city threatened to shut down emergency services. The report concludes: "Unless the public role is related to the whole system, well-intentioned recommendations may only serve to dig the City deeper into an impossible situation."[72]

New York and Philadelphia:
A Tale of Two Cities

In 1975, New York City was also headed toward fiscal collapse. A budget crisis developed, predicated on national economic trends characterized as "stagflation," which represented a slowing, or stagnation of the national economy along with high rates of inflation. One of the key components of demand on the city budget was the New York City Health and Hospitals Corporation, or HHC. The HHC was an entity developed and incorporated in 1970 to consolidate and streamline the municipal hospitals. By 1972, with its budget deficit at $98.2 million, the HHC was described by the New York State Study Commission as a "financial disaster."[73] Headlines warned of impending financial doom almost daily.[74]

As New York City stared down bankruptcy in 1975 with its hospital corporation streamlining plan failing, a little further south on Interstate 95, the City of Philadelphia was contemplating its own fate. In some ways Philadelphia was similarly situated, albeit on a smaller scale.[75] There were several committees charged with examining other mechanisms of governance.[76] The profile of the care that was needed was changing from inpatient to ambulatory and long-term care.[77] Both cities' budgets had trouble keeping up with the demands and were facing deficits and potentially high tax increases. Both had labor unions as major constituents with significant political power. They faced problems of waste, corruption, inefficiency in their public hospitals, and the bad press that inevitably accompanies public institutions that are publicly failing. Both had convened a variety of blue-ribbon panels and commissions to attempt to root out the problems. Philadelphia undertook yet another study with its consultant, Medicon.[78] Medicon was asked to reevaluate the health needs of the citizens of the city, project future needs, and develop a plan sufficient to meet them. New York had already done this, based on the 1966 recommendations by the Piel Commission,[79] and had increased its ambulatory capacity, and decreased its acute care inpatient capacity.

Conclusions

Medicare and Medicaid were being implemented in all hospitals—public, voluntary, and nonprofit. The logic was that this should have helped PGH. But the national economy was in a slowdown, and state governments responded by decreasing and slowing payments in their Medicaid plans.[80] More Philadelphians became unemployed as jobs left the city. And supplemental payments, now included in the reimbursement formula for care delivered as part of the medical school educational mission, had not yet been instituted. This created significant financial and organizational tensions among the partner institutions. Layers of bureaucratic complexity froze decision-making, creating an organization that resisted addressing critical operational issues, in an operational fashion, resulting in paralyzing inaction. Further, PGH's partner institutions acquired new access to capital markets for tax-exempt financing by the nonprofit hospitals using the new Philadelphia Hospital Authority, which protected the city's bond rating during a fiscally troublesome period for all American cities. In its existing governance structure as a city entity, PGH would not have been able to provide the city with the same bond rating protection, effectively sidelining it from modernization. The economic period called "stagflation" effectively captured the mood and tone of those governing, as well as the governed.

The die had been cast. The Philadelphia General Hospital, once described by Dr. Charles Mills as "indestructible as the pyramids,"[81] was destined by fate and circumstance to become part of Philadelphia's storied history instead of its uncharted future.

Notes

1. Excerpted from a service rating done by an anonymous medical intern or resident. The copy, with identifying information omitted, was sent from the Director of Professional Services, and initialed "JPE," to Dr. Ed Cooper. UPC 56.4, Box 2, general correspondence file for grants and fellowships, University of Pennsylvania, PGH Archives. Dates are not discernible, but a date and time stamp shows "19__".

2. See Rosemary Stevens, *American Medicine and the Public Interest* (New Haven: Yale University Press, 1976), chapters 18-22, for general background on hospital financing of care; see Rosemary Stevens, *In Sickness and in Wealth: American Hospitals in the Twentieth Century* (New York: Basic Books, 1989), generally, but especially for a discussion on the development, implementation, and implications of Blue Cross reimbursement in chapter 7, and chapters 10, 11 and 12 on institutional complexity associated with government and reimbursement.

3. See John O'Donnell, *Commissioned to Serve: A History of the Hospitals and Higher Education Facilities Authority of Philadelphia, on the Occasion of its 25th Anniversary* (Philadelphia: The Vantage Center, 2000), 1-86.

4. Letter to Dr. Lewis Bluemle and Dr. Truman Schnabel from David Maxey, Esq., January 5, 1968. UPC 56.5, Box 1, University of Pennsylvania, PGH Archives. This letter also references an opening negotiation with the city on the subject of Medicare.

5. See other letters from Maxey to the university dated January 17, February 17, and May 16, 1968. UPC 56.5, Box 1, University of Pennsylvania, PGH Archives.

6. Letter from Maxey to Beers at the University of Pennsylvania, dated March 31, 1969. UPC 56.5, Box 1, University of Pennsylvania PGH Archives.

7. Letter to Charles Farrell from Alfred Beers, dated March 27, 1969. UPC 56.5, Box 1, University of Pennsylvania PGH Archives.

8. Letter to Alfred Beers from Charles Farrell, dated March 28, 1969. UPC 56.5, Box 1, University of Pennsylvania, PGH Archives.

9. Letter to Dean Gelhorn from David Maxey, dated January 21, 1969. UPC 56.5, Box 1, University of Pennsylvania, PGH Archives.

10. Letters to Edward Martin and Ernest Zeger from Alfred Beers, both dated June 23, 1969. UPC 56.5, Box 1, University of Pennsylvania, PGH Archives.

11. Letter to David Maxey from Alfred Beers, dated June 23, 1969. UPC 56.5, Box 1, University of Pennsylvania, PGH Archives.

12. See other correspondence from Maxey, Beers, Farrell, and Gelhorn. UPC 56.5, Box 1, University of Pennsylvania, PGH Archives.

13. See minutes from the Medical Staff Budget Committee, October 2, 1969. UPC 56.9, Box 2, University of Pennsylvania, PGH Archives.

14. Letter to Elton Barclay, PGH executive director, from Harvey Brodovsky, Acting co-coordinator, Jefferson Division, July 18, 1969. UPC 56.9, Box 2, University of Pennsylvania, PGH Archives. A similar letter was sent to Earl Perloff by Brodovsky, dated the same day.

15. See draft copy of the agreement, 1969. UPC 56.9, Box 2, University of Pennsylvania PGH Archives. Also see multiple correspondence with the Department of Health, Education and Welfare, as well as Blue Cross, to address related issues.

16. Ibid.

17. Letter to Barclay from Dr. Cates, February 12, 1969. UPC 56.9, Box 2, University of Pennsylvania, PGH Archives.

18. Letter to Barclay from Brodovsky, February 17, 1969. UPC 56.9, Box 2, University of Pennsylvania, PGH Archives.

19. Departmental Staff summary, October 8, 1971, 9:00 AM. UPC 56.45, Box 1, University of Pennsylvania, PGH Archives.

20. "Tate Contacts University Regarding PGH," *The Daily Pennsylvanian* 21, March 1969.

21. Ibid.

22. Letter to Charles Farrell from Alfred Beers, dated March 27, 1969, and letter to Alfred Beers from Charles Farrell, dated March 28, 1969. UPC 56.5, Box 1, University of Pennsylvania, PGH Archives.

23. Reports described in the Mayor's Committee on Municipal Health Services, *Report of the Mayor's Committee on Municipal Health Services* (Philadelphia, 1970), including the Kling Report, the Duane Report, and the Hubbard Report (described in this chapter). All offer various levels of description of PGH's physical decline.

24. O'Donnell, 21-22. Frankford Hospital eventually got its bond issue for the patient care wing through the Philadelphia Hospitals Authority. This occurred only after they were able to settle their contract with Blue Cross and demonstrate sufficient financial projections to satisfy authority requirements.

25. Ibid., 23.

26. Ibid., 26.

27. Ibid., 24.

28. Ibid., 25.

29. Ibid., 34-35.

30. Ibid., 30-31.

31. Ibid.

32. See oral history interview by author with Ernest Zeger, who discusses at length the concerns expressed by PGH and city officials regarding New York City's impending bankruptcy, Philadelphia, June 22, 2003. Also see Maria K. Mitchell, "Privatizing New York City's Public Hospitals: The Politics of Policy Making" (Ph.D. dissertation, The City University of New York, 1998).

33. O'Donnell, 31.

34. Ibid., 36.

35. Ibid., 47-50.

36. O'Donnell, 47-49. Also see correspondence from Hospitals Authority executive director Donald Cramp outlining the details of the Hahnemann issue, author's private archives.

37. See Julie Fairman and Joan Lynaugh, *Critical Care Nursing: A History* (Philadelphia: University of Pennsylvania Press, 1998), 22-43; Stevens, *In Sickness and in Wealth*, 216-219, 322-331.

38. See K.M. Ludmerer, *Time to Heal: American Medical Education from the Turn of the Century to the Era of Managed Care* (New York: Oxford University Press, 1999), 3-220.

39. Michael B. Katz, *In the Shadow of the Poorhouse: A Social History of Welfare in America* (New York: Basic Books, 1986); Stevens, *In Sickness and in Wealth*, 284-320; Stevens, *American Medicine and the Public Interest*, 417-541.

40. Katz, *In the Shadow of the Poorhouse*, 284-287; Michael B. Katz, *The Undeserving Poor: From the War on Poverty to the War on Welfare* (New York: Pantheon Books, 1989), 124-137.

41. I. Unger and D. Unger, *LBJ: A Life* (New York: John Wiley and Sons, 1999).

42. F.W. Blaisdell, "Development of the City-County (Public) Hospital," *Archives of Surgery* 129 (7, 1994): 760-764.

43. See Paul Starr, *The Social Transformation of American Medicine: The Rise of a Sovereign Profession and the Making of a Vast Industry* (New York: Basic Books, 1982), chapters 2 and 3.

44. E. Sparer, *Medical School Accountability in the Public Hospital: The University of Pennsylvania and the Philadelphia General Hospital* (Unpublished Report: Health Law Project, University of Pennsylvania, 1974).

45. Mayor's Committee on Municipal Health Services, *Report of the Mayor's Committee on Municipal Health Services* (Philadelphia: Mayor's Committee on Municipal Health Services, February 1970), 49.

46. See Sparer.

47. Ibid., 77.

48. See H.F. Dowling, *City Hospitals: The Undercare of the Underprivileged* (Cambridge, MA: Harvard University Press, 1982); and C.M. Rosenberg, "Social Class

and Medical Care in 19th-Century America: The Rise and Fall of the Dispensary" in *Sickness and Health in America: Readings in the History of Medicine and Public Health*, eds. J.W. Leavitt and R.L. Numbers (Madison: University of Wisconsin Press, 1974), 309-322.

49. Mayor's Committee on Municipal Health Services, *Report of the Mayor's Committee on Municipal Health Services*.

50. Dowling, chapters 2 and 5.

51. Maria K. Mitchell , "Privatizing New York City's Public Hospitals: The Politics of Policy Making" (Ph.D. dissertation, The City University of New York, 1998).

52. Mayor's Committee on Municipal Health Services, *Report of the Mayor's Committee on Municipal Health Services*.

53. Ibid., 41.

54. JRB Associates, *Impact of the Closing of Philadelphia General Hospital* (McLean, VA, 1979).

55. Ibid., 2.

56. Over the next 25 years, local leadership acted upon the charge to address the situation by convening a multitude of studies, task forces, panels, and blue-ribbon commissions to investigate PGH and its related relationships. The reports generated provide insights on the complex issues facing Philadelphia, highlighting deficiencies and proposing action. Reports include: Edward V. Sparer, *Medical School Accountability in the Public Hospital: The University of Pennsylvania and the Philadelphia General Hospital* (Unpublished report: Health Law Project , University of Pennsylvania, 1974); Mayor's Committee on Municipal Health Services, *Report of the Mayor's Committee on Municipal Health Services* (Philadelphia: Mayor's Committee on Municipal Health Services, February 1970); JRB Associates, *Impact of the Closing of Philadelphia General Hospital* (McLean, VA, 1979); Joint Committee of Board of Health and Board of Trustees Report, *Report of the Joint Committee of the Board of Health and PGH Board of Trustees to Consider the Responsibilities of the City of Philadelphia for Personal Health Services, including Care of the Chronically Ill and Aged, and the Role of the Philadelphia General Hospital with Respect to these Responsibilities* (Philadelphia, 1967); City of Philadelphia, *A Comprehensive Report on the Disposition of the Services of Philadelphia General Hospital, as well as the Establishment of the Philadelphia Nursing Home and New and Expanded Programs of the Philadelphia Department of Public Health* (Philadelphia, May 1978); Hospital Survey Committee, *Report and Recommendations of the Hospital Survey Committee with Respect to Alternatives for the Provision of Medical Care Now Rendered to the Citizens of Philadelphia at Philadelphia General Hospital* (Philadelphia, May 1972); Philadelphia Department of Public Health, *Comments and Analysis of Hospital Survey Committee Report on Philadelphia General Hospital of May 2, 1972* (Philadelphia, May 1972); and Medicon Study, *Philadelphia General Hospital Final Report Preliminary Planning, Program of Requirements and Cost Estimates* (Philadelphia, 1976).

57. H. Levins, "Survey After Survey, and Yet No Action," *Philadelphia Daily News*, January 29, 1976, 19.

58. Mayor's Committee on Municipal Health Services, 43.

59. Ibid., 44.

60. Ibid., 45.

61. Ibid.

62. Ibid., 46.

63. Ibid., 46-47.

64. Ibid., 48.

65. Ibid.

66. Sparer, 36-51.

67. Ibid., 76-86.

68. H. Levins, "City Slowly Strangling Hospital, Says Staff," *Philadelphia Daily News*, January 30, 1976.

69. Mayor's Committee on Municipal Health Services, 49.

70. Ibid., 49. Also see a copy of the original report in the Polk private archives, Barbara Bates Center for Nursing History, University of Pennsylvania.

71. Mayor's Committee on Municipal Health Services, 92.

72. Ibid., 51; Sparer, 46-51. Also see the many articles in the *Philadelphia Daily News* that detail the changing demographics of the PGH patients.

73. Mitchell, 54-59.

74. Ibid., 47-62.

75. See oral history interview by author with Ernest Zeger, executive director of the PGH at the time of the closure, who asserts that New York City's fiscal problems were very much on the minds of those involved in trying to address the issues that PGH was facing, Philadelphia, June 22, 2003.

76. See Mitchell, 47-50, which outlines a number of blue ribbon panels and commissions focused on the governance and administration of the New York City public hospitals.

77. Mayor's Committee on Municipal Health Services, 48-50.

78. This study, commissioned less than a year before the closure announcement was made, was not completed. The study process was converted instead into a phase-out and a transition plan.

79. Mitchell, 48-54.

80. See oral history interview of Hillel Levinson, who describes the problems the city had in securing their Pennsycare payments during the administration of Governor Milton Shapp, Philadelphia, February 19, 2004.

81. Charles K. Mills, "The Philadelphia Almshouse and Philadelphia Hospital from 1854-1908," in *The History of Blockley*, ed. John Welsh Croskey (Philadelphia: F.A. Davis, 1929), 66.

5

The Closure:
The Beginning of the End

In January 1976, the movement to close Philadelphia General Hospital was gaining momentum. At the same time, the staff and management of the hospital continued to discuss and plan for alternative strategies for the ailing hospital. In a meeting of the Executive Committee on January 14, 1976, Dr. Patrick Storey discussed the five key "major trends taking place" at PGH, including planning for construction of a new hospital and exploring new forms of governance, in addition to other areas of planning for change.[1] In a meeting of the Joint Conference Committee on January 19, Tina Weintraub, executive director of PGH, announced that the consulting group Medicon had been selected to develop the PGH West project, one of the projects under consideration for replacing the antiquated physical plant. Weintraub also discussed the possibility of establishing something called Blockley Health Associates as a vehicle for contracting services between the city and the medical schools.[2]

The Movement to Closure Begins

PGH had problems on many fronts, including ones that found expression on the front pages of major Philadelphia newspapers. There was a continuing and significant nursing shortage at PGH, despite the presence of its own nursing school,[3] that resulted in the reduction of beds in both the medical intensive care unit and the cardiac care unit. The nursing shortage was reported in dramatic terms by the *Philadelphia Daily News*, whose front page headline on January 26, 1976, read, "PGH: Death by Neglect. . . Supply, Staff Shortages Killing Patients."[4]

In the article, several PGH physicians were quoted directly and on the record regarding poor care at PGH. Dr. Sandy Pomerantz, a PGH resident, said, "I had a patient die on me because there were no nurses available to take care of him." Dr. Robert Narins, a nationally known renal expert at PGH, stated, "It is not an exaggeration to say that a patient coming to PGH has a better chance of dying than if he went to another hospital."[5] An unnamed registered nurse was quoted as saying, "What you see could be called 'nigger medicine.'"[6]

That headline began a succession of articles by the *Philadelphia Daily News*, led in substantial part by a controversial reporter, Hoag Levins. Levins, who posed as a sick homeless alcoholic to gain admission to PGH, wrote a devastating series of articles, which included a detailed and horrifying portrait of the care he received during his undercover assignment. Day after day, these news stories, replete with direct quotes from PGH staff—some on the record, some off the record—painted a demoralizing portrait of a once-respected and honorable institution.

On January 27, 1976, the *Daily News* headline read, "PGH: Shortage of Nurses Endangers Patients."[7] The article detailed the absence of registered nurses for patient assignments on multiple specialty wards and on weekends. It also reported that on some units there were no registered nurses scheduled for up to 16 hours. Levins cited a three-month undercover investigation as the basis for the allegations, further alleging that PGH was not meeting minimum standards set by federal and state government. Levins anonymously quoted one nurse who left PGH, saying, "I left because I couldn't stand it anymore. I was going 100 miles an hour all the time, and still falling behind."[8] He asserted that due to horrendous working conditions, nurses left often, and PGH was forced to hire "rejects." In a related article in the same issue, Levins reported that PGH management engaged in a "nurse juggling act" to hide the shortage from the Department of Health, Education and Welfare, which sent representatives for an inspection based on complaints it had received.[9] He noted for the record that despite repeated phone calls, none of the PGH management would respond to inquiries made for the story.

The negative publicity continued. On January 28, the front page of the *Daily News* carried the headline "Inside PGH," featuring another devastating article and undercover photos taken of inadequate bathroom facilities, with as few as two toilets for 40 patients, and groups of patients sitting in wheelchairs in a hallway, which served as their lounge in the absence of proper facilities. Most damning, however, were comments from many PGH employees, on and off the record, who described horrendous patient care conditions, including rusted grapefruit juice cans serving as foley bags for urine collection in the absence of sufficient supplies; single, dirty bathtubs used for dozens of patients; poor lighting; no access to medical files after business hours; pediatric patients all housed in a large room, not separated by age as required by law; poor ventilation throughout the hospital; pharmacy access closed after 5 p.m.; and many other complaints.[10] In the same issue of the newspaper, an article titled "PGH Chairman Sells to His Own Hospital" identified Earl Perloff as a vendor to PGH. Although the reporter noted that Perloff did not violate the ethics code since the procurement department, not the hospital, was the contracting agency, the clear intimation was that Perloff had been less than ethical in his dealings as the chairman of the faltering institution.[11] The reporter also noted that Tina Weintraub, the executive director of PGH, and Dr. Lewis Polk, the acting health commissioner, had not returned any of the phone calls placed over the previous 10 days.

On the next day, January 29, the *Daily News* ran a photo of reporter Hoag Levins, posing as an "ailing derelict," lying on a PGH stretcher during his admission as a patient. The opening line of the accompanying article was uttered by a PGH staff member regarding Levins, the derelict patient poseur: "Hurry up and get that stinking son of a bitch out of here." In the most provocative article of the series, Levins described the less-than-humane care by staff and deplorable patient conditions, accompanied by pieces looking at the multiple studies commissioned on PGH and other alleged conflicting relationships with some of the people involved in one of the studies.[12]

On January 30, the *Daily News* asked "Is PGH Doomed?" in the headline of another extensive article. This piece focused on three areas: city employees suing the city to end the requirement that workers be treated at PGH; physicians who left PGH because of the poor conditions; and a study that analyzed budget cutbacks over a six-year period. In each piece, the failings of PGH to perform were highlighted in graphic terms.

The three city employees who brought the class action in Common Pleas Court asked the court to bar the city from requiring them to use PGH in order to qualify for "injured on duty" pay. According to their suit, being a patient at PGH was the only mechanism that would confer a set of benefits including full pay and free medical care. They cited the horrendous conditions at PGH as unacceptable and asked the court to restrain the city from forcing them to be cared for under these conditions. The suit named multiple members of the PGH leadership as defendants in the action.

Three PGH physicians—Dr. Robert Narins, the nationally renowned renal specialist; Dr. James Howard, who was chairman of a physician committee on patient care; and Dr. Les Dornfeld, chief of the dialysis unit at PGH—were also interviewed for this series. All had left PGH because of nursing and supply shortages that dramatically impacted their ability to practice. Each of them, on the record, spoke in compelling terms of their decisions to leave PGH.[13]

Finally, in a study conducted by the *Daily News*, an analysis of PGH budgets for the prior six years revealed dramatic drops in purchasing power in five of the six years, ranging from 6.8 to 9.8 percent, taking into account rates of inflation matched against budget increases (in '71, '73, and '74) or decreases (in '72 and '75). The study also reported significant decreases in patient admissions based on American Hospital Association data, which reported 18,607 admissions in 1971 compared to 13,325 in 1975.[14]

On Saturday, January 31, a *Daily News* headline screamed "Prosecution at PGH?" and reported that State Secretary of Health Leonard Bachman said that he might bring criminal charges against PGH officials if his staff discovered in their investigation that the officials had lied and covered up conditions at the hospital during a recent survey. Bachman went on to say that he had met with city Managing Director Hillel Levinson, who assured him the city would fully cooperate with the probe. In discussing the care of the poor of Philadelphia, Bachman stated, "If I was a poor person, I would go to a non-public hospital if I could."[15]

In the days that followed, the Philadelphia news outlets published story after story on the PGH failures. The *Philadelphia Tribune* reported that the National Association for the Advancement of Colored People (NAACP) made a formal request to the Department of Health, Education and Welfare to place PGH in receivership until "the deplorable conditions" had been corrected. Additional requests of the NAACP included a review of the PGH administration on account of the lack of African Americans on the board or in any leadership posts.[16] On February 3, a *Daily News* editorial urged action by the city and the state, ending with the demand, "Either close the place and stop killing people, or do something."[17] The same day, 42 staff physicians called for action at PGH, openly planning to divert patients to area hospitals in order to ensure proper care.[18] In the same issue, columnist Chuck Stone commended his intrepid fellow journalist, saying, "This past December, my blond, blue-eyed colleague, Hoag Levins, became a nigger. By blackening his face? Easier than that. Simply by entering the Philadelphia General Hospital as a patient. . . Levins [is] one of this nation's brightest reportorial stars."[19] On February 10, Levins reported that the state knew about the nursing shortage, but did little.[20] On February 11, the *Daily News* reported that the Joint Commission on the Accreditation of Hospitals (JCAH) was beginning an unscheduled inspection of PGH that day, in response to the exposé. While the unscheduled visit would last several days, the findings would not be reported until sometime in March or April, after being reviewed by the entire commission in Chicago.[21]

Inside PGH

Meanwhile, the negative publicity was finding expression in the internal workings of PGH. On February 6, in a letter addressed to the Executive Committee, Dr. Sheila Murphy, chairperson of the Patient Care Committee, urgently requested that the job freeze[22] that had been implemented at PGH be eliminated, and all approved budget expenditures be implemented as soon as possible, stating, "The present practice which refuses to purchase approved items or supplies by interminable bureaucratic delay or outright refusal to spend allocated funds is grossly irresponsible and must be stopped. A hospital requires supplies and equipment in order to function. The [Patient Care] Committee considers that the above requests represent merely the minimum, bare essentials of our needs. Failure to meet these requests will eventually destroy our ability to function as a hospital."[23] Murphy concluded the letter by writing, "The Committee realized that PGH faces many problems in both the near and distant future whose solutions remain unclear. However, we feel that the above recommendations must be implemented soon if we are to have a future."[24]

On February 9, a special session of the Executive Committee was called. Executive Director Tina Weintraub notified those assembled that due to the negative publicity regarding PGH, JCAH would be coming to Philadelphia for a three-day inspection, beginning the day after next. Weintraub openly protested the inspection since PGH would also be under review by the Professional Standards Review Organization on those days, and the overtime budget was already straining the resources of the institution. JCAH was not persuaded and the inspection commenced.[25]

On February 11, the Executive Committee met and the letter from Dr. Murphy of the Patient Care Committee was read into the record, and endorsed by the Executive Committee, with the proviso that the letter be forwarded to the Board of Trustees for their meeting on February 19. The report of medical director Patrick Storey opened with the start of the JCAH survey, which commenced that morning. Dr. Storey informed the Executive Committee that one member of the inspecting team held an open, two-hour meeting with the house staff and three members of the Department of Medicine. In this meeting, the multiple inadequacies of PGH were cited by the medical staff, which recommended that the accreditation of PGH be rescinded. Dr. Storey put the question to the body: Should they endorse this approach as a solution? He asked the committee to consider, "What is the advantage to the hospital of having its accreditation revoked?"[26]

Throughout the meeting of the Executive Committee, multiple points of view were expressed regarding the actions of various physician groups and individuals who formed the medical staff and house staff. Dr. Howard Hurting said that the dissident house staff believed that they were making constructive efforts, not destructive efforts, to help the hospital. Dr. Edward Cooper voiced confidence in the physicians who were leaders in the effort, calling them "the most responsible, capable core persons of his group." Both Dr. Gladys M. Miller and Dr. Storey were on the record noting that the lack of trust between the two physician groups—attendings and house staff—created a problem among the physicians and prevented a unified approach. One physician pointed out that, even as they were speaking, house staff was handing out leaflets to patients at the entrances of PGH, encouraging them to attend a public meeting later that week. When no consensus could be reached, another meeting was called for on Monday, February 16, which would include the entire medical staff.[27]

The Closure Announcement

On February 15, 1976, a final decision was reached. Managing Director Hillel Levinson announced that PGH would close within the next year.[28] The announcement was preceded by a series of internal phone calls to alert key staff. Initially, Levinson asked Dr. Lewis Polk to make the announcement. Polk refused, leaving Levinson to issue the press release himself.[29] Ernest Zeger, the assistant executive director, called Director of Nursing Stephanie Stachniewicz to inform her the day before the announcement was made. Stachniewicz professed shock since she had been playing an active role in planning for the new hospital that was to be constructed.[30] She, like Polk, believed that it was a bad decision that would not be well received by many key PGH constituencies.

On the following day, February 16, at what was to have been a meeting for the medical staff to discuss how to unify their efforts to rectify PGH, the entire medical staff issued a joint public statement that said they "take the strongest exception to the precipitous decision to close the PGH."[31] The statement went on to discuss and predict "disastrous consequences," and their belief that the closure was "illegal, contravening both the City Charter and Federal Regulations." On February 17, a demonstration of about 200 individuals representing three different advocate groups was held at City Hall.[32] Mayor Rizzo, in an impromptu interview outside his office, said the decision was "final" and that "nothing will turn it around."[33] The same day, union leaders representing more than 2,000 PGH employees called for a protest the following week.[34] The following day, City Council members weighed in. Council President George Schwartz asked the mayor for a meeting between members of the administration and City Council. Schwartz described the closure as "premature," and said that "insufficient study has been made. Proper arrangements with other hospitals have not been made. . . ," and Councilwoman Ethel Allen, the only physician member of City Council, also expressed concerns.[35]

In another internal matter that quickly became public, the PGH Board of Trustees, many of whom were angered that they were not kept apprised of the decision-making within the city administration, reacted. In a February 18 letter to Mayor Rizzo, the chairman of the board, Earl Perloff, tendered his resignation, effective immediately, saying, "I cannot and should not be asked to participate in the dissolution of this once proud institution, which has been permitted to deteriorate through a consistent pattern of budgetary under-financing and a failure to make meaningful capital improvements."[36]

That same day, another special meeting of the PGH Executive Committee was called to discuss the implications of the now-officially-announced closure. Most of the discussion focused on the significant problems associated with the intern/resident matching program, the potential collapse of the program, and all of the attendant ramifications, which included the imminent departure of acute care patients, such that the house staff under contract would seek employment elsewhere. Other issues raised included the absorption of non-tenured staff; how to cope with the panic of the precipitous announcement; priorities of essential services; the training program underway, commitments already made for the following year, and the need to contract for certain services in the coming year.[37]

At this meeting, there was also a discussion of the statement that had been issued earlier in the day by the hospital medical staff. Dr. Austen Sumner, who expected to be interviewed on Channel 3 television, wished to use the statement as a guide in answering an editorial. Representatives from the house staff took exception to paragraph five of the statement, which read, "Our patients cannot be cared for elsewhere, and we believe that they will suffer if PGH closes. We reject the recent claims that medical care at PGH is poor. This hospital has always offered a high level of care, and continues to do so."[38] Dr. Charles Heaton informed the objecting house staff that the statement, as written, had been endorsed by the Board of Trustees, the Executive Committee, the Nursing Department, and the union. Dr. Sumner was then given the clearance to use the statement. The board further voted and agreed that the statement should be published in its entirety in the *Sunday Bulletin* and the *Philadelphia Tribune*.[39]

The statement of the physician group was the first that questioned the legality of the decision to close PGH. But other questions, in other venues of inquiry, quickly followed.

Reaction to the Closure

On February 20, representatives of seven other city hospitals asked for a meeting with the city administration to discuss the increased burden they would face as a result of the closure. At the same time, City Council President Schwartz criticized the administration for their lack of consultation regarding the closure. The same day, the state Superior Court upheld the order of Common Pleas Court Judge Eugene Gelfand, who had issued a restraining order forbidding the city from taking any further action pending a hearing on the closure. This was pursuant to a suit filed by Charles Bowser, a former mayoral opponent of Frank Rizzo. Bowser filed the suit on behalf of PGH physicians Cynthia Cook and Richard Freeman, several PGH patients, and Rev. James Preston, president of the Baptist Ministers Conference of Philadelphia and Vicinity. The suit charged that PGH could not be closed without an amendment to the City Charter.[40]

On February 21, the African-American political community stepped into the fray. State Representative David Richardson called for a full legislative investigative hearing on PGH. The NAACP, led by regional director Jerry Guess, threw its support behind a demonstration scheduled with PGH union members the following week.[41] The next day, City Councilwoman Ethel Allen announced her intention to offer an alternative proposal to the closure. Allen, a Republican, outlined the proposed elements of her bill, saying, "I intend to develop this bill so carefully that no one can dispute its logic. With Judge Gelfand's injunction barring the City from interrupting or curtailing any PGH services, I will have time to do that."[42]

But the court reprieve was short-lived. Two days later, Common Pleas Judge G. Fred DiBona lifted the temporary restraining order, ruling that the city was not legally required to maintain a public hospital. Attorney Charles Bowser stated that he would appeal and declined to put on witnesses to support the argument that the decision was "capricious," saying, "There is no point in proceeding before this judge."[43] At the hearing, Edward Sparer, a law professor at the University of Pennsylvania, unsuccessfully argued the case,[44] where more than 100 supporters of PGH crowded the courtroom.[45]

That same day, other wheels were in motion. Mayor Rizzo met with members of City Council to explain the reasons that the administration was pursuing the closing and described the plan to phase out the hospital. Earl Stout, the president of District Council 33, announced that day that the union was calling a one-day "holiday" so that city workers could join in the protest rally against the city administration's plans to close PGH. [46]

Protest and Recall

On February 25, 2,500 people marched to City Hall to protest the closure. After some confusion about the starting time, the march began with protest songs and signs in the air. The march, which started at the front door of PGH and culminated at City Hall, was led by union leaders and patients in wheelchairs. Addressing those assembled from the back of a flatbed truck, Charles Bowser said of the mayor's decision to close PGH: "It's one word—recall." The crowd began to chant: "Recall, recall, recall. . . ."[47]

The following day, the Regional Comprehensive Planning Council discussed the PGH closure. The proposal from Councilwoman Allen calling for the preservation of a modified version of PGH that kept intact the school of nursing was acknowledged.[48] But the situation was described as "too fluid" to draw any conclusions as to the outcome.[49]

On February 27, City Council members Joseph Coleman, Earl Vann, and Cecil B. Moore addressed the closure at a regularly scheduled council meeting. Coleman asked, and Vann and Moore insisted, that the mayor should hold a public meeting to explain the administration's reasons for desiring the closure. These same councilmen had previously announced their intention to launch an investigation into the conditions at PGH when the closure was announced. "Maybe the public will have a better idea," said Coleman, who chaired the council's standing committee on public health and welfare.[50]

At a raucous City Council meeting less than two weeks later, members tried to advance the PGH case. Councilman Lucien Blackwell introduced a resolution calling for hearings. Council President George Schwartz, offering no comment on his position, said that Blackwell's resolution "would be referred to an appropriate committee." Councilwoman Allen rose to speak to the fact that she had not yet been provided with any information regarding the city's plans to cope with the ramifications of the closure. "I have yet to see such plans," said Allen, who then addressed her colleagues, saying, "Within the next three to four weeks, the interns at PGH will have to decide whether or not to seek other jobs. . . Unless we act soon, it will be much too late to save the hospital." None of her fellow council members reacted or responded to her entreaties.[51] The lack of reaction, by City Council as a body and by President Schwartz, signaled that there would likely be no public hearings, since there was an uneasy truce between Rizzo and Schwartz, who was being careful not to strain the already tenuous relationship.[52]

Turmoil and Transition

The leadership of PGH had to cope with the operation of the hospital while political machinations continued, and arguments for either directional change or closure were advanced. These competing arguments made for difficult management of an unstable, and unpredictable, situation.

In the weeks and months that followed, the complexities of coping with a hospital in turmoil faced key constituencies of PGH. There were many people in significant roles of responsibility who had little or no sense of how the closure would proceed, or even if it would proceed at all.[53] While the hospital's functioning was described as "business as usual," the management of PGH spiraled into chaos. At the next meeting of the Board of Trustees on March 16, Acting Health Commissioner Polk was to present a status report along with significant information and agenda items that required board action, but the meeting was so poorly attended that there was no quorum, and the business of the board could not be completed.[54] At this meeting, Polk disclosed figures demonstrating that earlier estimates of the number of patients being served by PGH were inflated.[55] Using these revised numbers, Polk asserted that there would be no significant strain on other hospitals to absorb too heavy an increased patient load. In addition, Polk offered assurances that there had been no "shenanigans" in billing practices, and that the executives for both Blue Cross and the Medicaid program, Bruce Taylor and Glen Johnson, were on record that they believed they had not been improperly billed for reimbursed services.

While "business as usual" was billed as the modus operandi at the hospital, it was clear that the turmoil was having a significant internal impact. At the medical staff cabinet meeting on March 4, Dr. Charles Heaton, president of the medical staff, insisted that it was important that "we continue all functions, meetings and activities appropriate to an accredited institution."[56] In the course of the meeting, other committee chairs noted significant closure-related problems. House Staff Committee Chair Dr. Gladys Miller stated that plans regarding the house staff are "on a state of chaos." Patient Care Committee Chair Dr. Sheila Murphey informed the committee that the effect of the closure announcement on the recruitment of nurses and house staff "has been catastrophic."[57] This is especially noteworthy since PGH was already suffering from a nursing shortage.

On April 1, 1976, Dr. Heaton announced at the medical staff cabinet meeting that Executive Director Tina Weintraub had submitted her resignation, with Ernest Zeger succeeding her as acting executive director. In his remarks to the cabinet, Zeger noted that there was a continuing community effort to save the hospital, and that funds had been appropriated to keep the hospital open for the next year.[58] In later years, Zeger recalled that it was not clear in the early months following the closure announcement that the hospital would, in fact, close.[59] This was echoed in remarks made by Dr. Heaton at a later meeting, where he stated that the matter of the PGH closing was not a "dead issue yet."[60]

The lack of PGH utilization and the implications that the closure would not be difficult to achieve began to seep into the public consciousness. *Philadelphia Inquirer* medical writer Donald Drake, in an extensive analysis piece, wrote: "Looking at the sprawling complex of PGH buildings, it's hard to believe that other existing hospitals could absorb the patients handled by such a large facility. But in this case, looks are deceiving. . . Take, as an example, the inpatient census of March 1st." Drake goes on to note that although PGH was built to accommodate 2,000 patients, on that day the hospital had only 918 beds available. Of that 918, only 688 beds were filled and only 202 of those patients were classified as "acutely ill." Of the remaining 486, many were "disposition problems," and Drake estimated that only about 300 patients would actually need ongoing hospitalization in acute care beds. These figures roughly coincide with Polk's analysis, in which he said that of the average daily census of 500 patients at PGH, approximately half were nursing home cases.[61]

The public discussion regarding the closure continued with consternation and speculation on various fronts. There was ongoing public dissatisfaction with the slow release of a cogent plan for closure and transfer of hospital services. More than five weeks after the announcement, there was mounting concern that multiple patient groups were still without a thoughtful resolution as to how they might be cared for, including addicted pregnant women; "neurologic cripples," mostly victims of gang violence and accidents; rape victims, which numbered about a thousand cases a year; victims of child abuse; city employees; psychiatric patients, including detox patients; and dental patients, which constituted approximately 8,000 visits annually. Each of these patient categories represented a unique set of problems and issues that had to be addressed.[62]

In almost every exchange, the fiscal demand of PGH on the city's overall financial health was cited. In 1975, the noncapital operating budget of PGH was $44.6 million. Fringe benefits for employees, at a cost of $5.7 million, were paid for out of the city's general fund, not out of the PGH budget. About $27.6 million came from state and federal government reimbursements, leaving the city with $17 million in additional funds it needed to generate, most of which came from city tax revenues.[63]

On April 20, at a meeting of City Council, President George Schwartz expressed ongoing dissatisfaction that the mayor's administration had still not provided a clear plan for the closing. "We expected a white paper from the administration with a detailed plan. . . it has not been forthcoming," Schwartz complained.[64] The other members of City Council, including Dr. Ethel Allen, Lucien Blackwell, Joseph Coleman, and Cecil B. Moore—all of whom were African American—joined him in his sentiments. At the same meeting, Acting Health Commissioner Lewis Polk informed the council members that although there were no written agreements with any area hospitals, representatives of those hospitals "seemed to agree" that they would be able to care for the PGH patients that would be displaced by the closing.[65]

The Administration Responds

A week later, on April 28, Managing Director Hillel Levinson wrote to Council President George Schwartz: "As I promised you last week during the operating budget hearings, I am sending you this day the first of several administration reports on Philadelphia General Hospital, along with copies of the latest consultant's report. . . .Copies of each of these documents are included for all of the members of Council."[66] In the letter, Levinson pointed out that PGH received accreditation from the Joint Commission on the Accreditation of Hospitals for one year, which would assist the city in recouping reimbursements from care delivered during the phase-out period. He also reasserted that JCAH's conclusions regarding the physical plant issues at PGH further supported the administration's position that the "massive reconstruction and renovations [that] are necessary at PGH [would] make that course [non-closure] financially and practically unfeasible."[67]

The 15-page report, cited in the *Philadelphia Bulletin* the following day, summarized several issues (most of which were previously reported by numerous sources), and focused extensively on the severely deteriorated condition of the facility and the substantial costs associated with either refurbishing or replacing the hospital. The article noted that all previous cost estimates were now much higher, since they had excluded inflation and financing, bringing the estimates from $105 million to over $200 million, excluding operating costs, which went from $7.5 million to $10 million annually.[68]

Most importantly, the report cited 1975 statistics demonstrating that on an average day there were 1800 empty general hospital beds in Philadelphia, seven times the number needed for patients served by PGH in an acute care setting. It further asserted that "the proposed plan will afford equal opportunity for all of our citizens to receive the same quality care in the hospital and neighborhood of their choice, and eliminate the stigma of being cared for in a charity institution," which in many instances can be distant and difficult to reach. The voluntary hospitals assured the city that they could accommodate the acute inpatient load from PGH, and in doing so bring down their present bed vacancies. A spokesman for a group of the area hospitals, including the bulk of the institutions most likely to be affected, said in a March 1 news release that "their hospitals were willing and able to care for those patients ordinarily admitted to acute care to PGH" and they "agreed that Philadelphia hospitals have enough beds [without PGH] to care for the acutely ill."[69]

The report went on to explain the benefits of renovating the former Landis Hospital to become a skilled and intermediate care facility. Under this new approach, the city would receive enhanced reimbursements due to changes in the reimbursement formula, and the level of care would be appropriate to the needs of the patients.

Patients who needed ongoing care would be transferred from PGH to Landis when the renovations were complete.

Addressing another area of concern, the city outlined a plan to expand the existing outpatient services available in the city's district health centers. Based on their analysis of the geography of the outpatient visits provided at PGH and the existing health centers, outpatient visits would be transferred to the district clinic facilities that are more "geographically convenient" for the patients.[70] The plan included $835,000 in the FY 1977 capital budget for the upgrading of district health centers to accommodate the new demands.

The report also acknowledged that "the administration recognizes the inadequacy of the reimbursements for outpatient and emergency care by the State Medicaid Program. The administration has pledged its support to the voluntary hospitals of our city in their continuing struggle to increase these reimbursements to a level approaching reasonable costs. Toward this end, the City Administration has made contacts with the Governor and is supporting appropriate legislation proposed by the voluntary hospitals through their state association."[71]

Other PGH programs were listed, with individual commentary as to the status of either its phase-out, including the schools of medical technology and X-ray; or plans for relocation, as with the Center for Rape Concerns and the Child Abuse Center, in which preliminary discussions with other hospitals were being conducted to ensure transfer of "viable programs" with "hospitals that have expressed an interest."[72]

The report concluded: "To sum up, the City Administration believes that it has insured and will insure the delivery of vital services throughout the transition period and into the future. . . It is not an easy task to make such a major change, even one that is so obviously necessary as phasing out the obsolete Philadelphia General Hospital buildings and the revitalization of the health care programs. The partners in the PGH project—the City and the voluntary hospitals—recognize this responsibility, and, working together, will make the phase-out a success."[73]

Wheels in Motion

At a City Council hearing on April 29, Council President Schwartz read aloud a letter from Hillel Levinson that asserted the intention of the administration to reassign 86 hospital laundry employees, most of whom were District Council 33 members, after the laundry facility was sold. The letter was followed by a public assertion by Schwartz that he would actively oppose the sale unless assurances were given that the workers would be placed in other city jobs. The administration had been seeking the sale of the laundry unit but had been stymied in its intentions. City Council, in a 10-4 vote, approved the bill.[74]

As the meetings and deliberations continued, a gradual shift in the tone of some of the key constituencies began to emerge. On May 2, the *Philadelphia Bulletin* reported the apparent "softening of their [the voluntary hospitals'] position," which had been previously described as predicting "financial disaster" for their institutions. Representatives from most of the seven area hospitals went on the record in the article, reiterating their intention to cooperate and partner with the city in respect to the closure of PGH and the transfer of patients, present and future, into their respective institutions. This change in tone "came after some hard looks at the facts and a couple of jaw-boning sessions with city officials."[75] The following day, the president of the Delaware Valley Hospital Association, representing its 43 member hospitals, issued a statement that city-based hospitals would need additional financial assistance, from the $2 million they currently received to $5 million annually, in order to function with the new level of demand. He stated, "Hospitals cannot survive under a prolonged, piecemeal system for corrective action. Reimbursement at reasonable cost for out-patient emergency service remains a vital need at the governmental level."[76]

Meanwhile, the staff conditions at PGH continued to deteriorate. In a meeting of the medical staff Executive Committee, the physicians assembled expressed concern that they would not have enough flexibility or staff to manage the ongoing operational difficulties. Dr. Sheila Murphey announced that because of the "precipitous announcement of closing PGH," they were unable to recruit enough house staff to continue to run a large acute care facility. Dr. William Long requested that the assembled group act to adopt recommendations that would permit the physicians in charge to exercise a higher level of discretion in accepting admissions and managing patient flow. Ernest Zeger announced that the city had decided not to accept another class of nursing students in the fall, a decision that "was met with great concern on the part of our Executive Committee, since the school has had a very long and illustrious history."[77] Other physicians expressed dissatisfaction with the Medicon study, questioning the validity of their data.[78]

On May 4, local union leadership announced that 300 international union officials would come to Philadelphia later in the month to hold a national conference on the issue of saving public hospitals. Al Johnson, president of Local 488 of the American Federation of State, County and Municipal Employees (AFSCME), and Jay Kogan, president of AFSCME Council 47, held a news conference where they made this announcement, and also called for a march to protest the closure on May 22.[79]

Internally, the hospital leadership continued to struggle with the media accounts that were driving public perceptions. During an Executive Committee meeting on May 12, the members debated whether or not to employ someone for the express purpose of managing the public relations issues that the hospital was facing as a direct result of the almost daily battering PGH was taking in the Philadelphia papers. In a spirited discussion about allocation of limited resources, actual costs, political implications, and misperceptions of image related to the disbursement funds for public relations staff, the committee agreed to approve a contract for public relations consulting on a month-to-month basis.

The following day, the *Philadelphia Daily News* began a series of analysis pieces in which the litany of grievances regarding the failure of PGH and its leadership was recited. In these stories, Hoag Levins challenged the credibility of everyone involved with the management and administration of PGH. Levins noted that "Some opposition to closing has developed and another protest is scheduled for May 22nd. But the opponents appear to be weak. There seems little doubt the hospital will close. Most of the opposition is coming from hospital employees who are more worried about their jobs than the quality of care available to the City's poor. A few other critics who demanded better care. . . now seem to be primarily concerned about saving PGH as a last resort for the poor—regardless of the quality of care."[80]

The final protest march against the closing was held on May 22 with 500 demonstrators, made up mostly of union members and patients in wheelchairs. A hearse led the march with six "pallbearers" carrying a sign saying "This Might Be Your Next Ride If PGH Closes." They marched from the hospital to Independence Hall, where several leaders of constituent groups spoke to the marchers and curious tourists. They called on those assembled to "bombard their councilmen with protests over the proposed closing."[81]

On June 9 in a Medical Executive Committee meeting, Ernest Zeger announced that the city would finalize a lease agreement that morning with the Commonwealth of Pennsylvania for the Landis Hospital for $1 yearly, commencing on June 22. This was a critical component in the city's plan to transfer the "disposition cases" to a skilled nursing facility. Now that this important piece was in place, the city and PGH staff could proceed with the transition plan.[82] Zeger discussed in detail some of the steps that would be necessary, including the "unfreezing" of 60 to 70 positions by the Managing Director's office to complete the phase-out in an orderly fashion. Other members of the committee decried the ongoing personnel shortage and the severe morale problems that were besetting the day-to-day function of the hospital.[83]

Despite ongoing public criticism,[84] the closure/transition plan continued to move forward. On August 13, 1976, the Commonwealth Court handed the city administration the final approval that they had been waiting for by upholding the lower court ruling and rejecting a suit by citizens' groups seeking to block the city from closing PGH. In its decision, the court wrote: "The thrust of the appellant's arguments is that the more than 200 year history of statutes authorizing a hospital for the indigent in Philadelphia creates a duty upon the City to continue to maintain PGH. . . It is a novel argument for which we find no precedent."[85] The opinion went on to say that the mayor had the power to reject expenditures, and also rejected the argument that the state, not the city, had the power to close the facility.[86] With this court ruling, the city government faced no further legal or structural impediments to the closing of PGH. The end of an era had come, and a most extraordinary institution was soon to pass into historic memory.

The Long Goodbye

Over the next several months, PGH functions and services were moved as various contracts and agreements were finalized. By September 1976, all of the outpatient services were transferred to district health centers around the city. Maternity care services and the rape treatment program were closed and transferred to four contract hospitals.[87] Maternity care would now be provided as part of the Family Medical program and contracting hospitals would perform the delivery. The new rape program was to be coordinated by Women Organized Against Rape, a local nonprofit organization. Deputy Health Commissioner Lawrence Devlin announced that the city had executed a contract with Hahnemann Hospital to fill the gaps of physician coverage during the transition of the new program, which was expected to take up to six months.[88]

As these core services were being closed, some individuals still committed to the concept of an enduring PGH refused to stand down. On September 8, at a PGH Executive Committee meeting, Dr. Alan Steinberg proposed that the committee go on record as being willing to revitalize all of the services that had formerly been offered by PGH if the decision to close the hospital was reversed. The Executive Committee voted unanimously in favor of Steinberg's proposal.[89] The PGH chaplain, Rev. Robert Lee Maffett, continued to press the community to stand up for PGH. He pushed for a recall of Mayor Rizzo, passing out voter registration cards to vote Rizzo out by supporting the recall effort. But when the Pennsylvania Supreme Court ruled that the recall action was unconstitutional, "It was like doomsday among the people [at PGH]," said Chaplain Maffett. Maffett said he still refused to give up.[90]

At the time of the closure announcement, it was estimated that PGH's inpatient load had dropped from 1,858 in 1960 to 800, largely due to Medicare, Medicaid, and other health plan funding. Of those 800 patients, 400 would qualify as nursing home patients who, at that time, were expected to be fully covered by the Commonwealth. Of the non-nursing home patients, 200 could be transferred to other facilities since they had health plans that would cover their care. That left approximately 200 patients who would be more difficult placements, and included patients with drug and alcohol diagnoses, battered children, rape victims, and infectious disease cases, like tuberculosis. Philadelphia area hospitals noted that the greatest area of concern involved the absorption of the perceived huge ambulatory and emergency load of patients previously managed by PGH.[91]

The job of transitioning the patients, and effecting an orderly closing, would fall to many in the administration, some of whom

would be especially assigned out of other responsibilities in government. At the time of the closure announcement there were 40,000
outpatients and 400 emergency and acute patients.[92] Barry Savitz, a
young health center manager in the Department of Public Health,
was assigned to ensure that patient continuity was achieved. The district health centers would be responsible for managing the care of
PGH patients who could be discharged. The PGH physicians were
reassigned to the district health centers and the Family Medical program was established. This program provided continuing care for
PGH patients in an ambulatory setting. In what was a remarkable
feat even by today's standards, all PGH patients kept their own treating physicians.[93] This new program, which replaced "categorical
care" programs such as treatment of tuberculosis or venereal disease,
was a city-wide expansion of an existing comprehensive program
that received federal funds as part of a Model Cities project.[94]

    This newly implemented approach to ambulatory patient care
was more than a transition plan. It followed a partial fulfillment of a
1972 recommendation by the Hospital Survey Committee that the
City of Philadelphia convert the nine city-owned and operated district health centers into Neighborhood Ambulatory Care Centers.
The same report further recommended that the city construct two
new 200-bed acute care hospitals; that it purchase specialty medical
services from the affiliated medical school hospitals; and that it supply a total of 600 beds for chronic and long-term care.[95] But the new
direction emanating from the PGH closure, which included not
implementing plans for the construction of two smaller, more modern public hospitals, was clearly not the intent of the 1972 report.
The report highlighted the fact that many of the nonprofit hospitals
were facing significant fiscal challenges because of their care of large
groups of indigent patients.[96]

    These concerns continued to surface throughout the transition
period. On October 19, Mayor Rizzo held a lengthy meeting to reas-
sure doubtful members of City Council and others that indigent
patients would be cared for by private hospitals, and that no one
would be turned away from any hospital emergency room. After
extended discussions that covered the new plan for outpatient care
and contracts with city hospitals, City Council President George
Schwartz, historically skeptical of the administration's plans, con-
ceded, "The administration is on the right track."[97]

But not everyone was satisfied. In December, representatives of 41 community groups met with the Fellowship Commission to discuss their ongoing concerns that the poor would be left out. While the gathering could not agree on how they might play a role in addressing the problems that they anticipated with the closure, they agreed to continue to press the city for answers to the ongoing and emerging questions.[98]

Concurrently, PGH staff continued to face the realities of the dismantling of their institution. As more physicians left leadership roles on hospital committees, other physicians had to be recruited, with great difficulty, to fill in. It was increasingly problematic to maintain training for surgical residents because of the lack of patients, or "teaching material," since admissions had declined by 25 to 30 percent. The nursing shortage continued to grow worse. The rare book and periodical collections of the historic hospital had to be attended to, and arrangements had to be made for successor institutions to take receipt.[99]

The Final Days of PGH

Over the last six months of operation, the staff of PGH pressed on toward the closure, focusing on the necessary tasks, and considering a variety of options for addressing evolving issues. At the medical staff Executive Committee meeting in January 1977, issues surrounding the various historic PGH collections were considered, including the possibility of having a museum on the grounds. At the same time, the demands for the management of ongoing medical issues continued to occupy the attention of the medical staff, including audits of lab work, credentialing issues, the lack of autopsies for pathology interns and residents to conduct, and the staffing problems that continued as vacancies increased. As more PGH clinics continued to close and services transferred to other institutions, the medical staff focused on the details necessary to complete the execution of contracts, including issues related to malpractice coverage.[100]

Keeping the momentum going to run the institution and effectuate the closing at the same time presented significant challenges for PGH leadership. At the committee meeting in February, the Pharmacy and Therapeutic Committee requested by way of Stephanie Stachneiwicz, a member of the committee, that they be permitted to meet bimonthly. Charles Heaton, the committee chair, denied permission, saying that "monthly meetings must continue for as long as the hospital continues to function."[101] The need to address more than 900 incomplete patient charts was discussed, as were the ongoing plans and details associated with the transferring of the contingent of patients to Landis Hospital. There was agreement to continue to press the city to permit the medical staff to "help preserve the museum artifacts," and a discussion by the ad hoc committee on memorabilia that there were still many unsettled matters regarding the collections, noting, "No progress has been made."[102]

Final meetings of key committees that ran the internal operations of PGH were increasingly the order of the day. The Research and Publications Committee announced that they would hold no further monthly meetings. On March 10, the last meeting of the Hospital Radiation Safety Committee was held. Arrangements to transfer radioisotopes to another licensee and to schedule the last shipment of isotopes and final badge readings for each employee were made. Some committees were making arrangements to transfer their functions to the new nursing home. The Utilization Review Committee said they would continue to meet monthly, advising the Medical Staff Committee that the patients who were anticipated to go to the new nursing home were being consolidated in the Mills Building. So far, 150 patients had been transferred to Mills. The Medical Records Committee was authorizing a skeleton crew to finish copying records to transfer with patients.[103]

The final meeting of the medical staff Executive Committee was held on May 11, 1977. The Patient Care Committee reported that the hospital census was 94 and "transition going well."[104] In the minutes, the comments from the president read: "This is the last official Executive Committee meeting. Another will be called only if there are problems with memorabilia or some other department. During this month, the committees still required to meet are Patient Care Committee, Medical Records-Utilization Review Committee, Pharmacy and Therapeutics Committee, and Infection Control Committee. Dr. Gibbons [the newly named medical director of the nursing home unit] is to be contacted when these meetings occur."[105] At the conclusion of the meeting, Dr. Heaton was thanked for his leadership and given a standing ovation.[106]

During that period, the press coverage of the closure indicated the almost anticlimactic nature of the final days of PGH. Most of the activity centered on finalization of necessary contracts; full implementation of the family medical program; the delineation of chronic patients who would transfer to Landis Hospital, which would later become the Philadelphia Nursing Home; and the transfer of PGH employees into other types of city roles.[107] But there were moments when the historical significance for those involved with this once noble institution was overwhelming.

The graduation of the final class of PGH nurses was one of those moments. The nurses, who were educated in the tradition of Alice Fisher to wear the double frill cap as a symbol of nursing care excellence, said a sad goodbye to the PGH School of Nursing on June 10, 1977, as the last graduating class of 72 new nurses departed. Over the 92-year history of the school, 6,000 nurses graduated from "Old Blockley," as the school was affectionately known. Eileen (Duffy) Kelly, the president of the last graduating class, said that the student body was informed that the hospital would close the day after the School of Nursing graduation. Said Kelly, "[We felt] anger, hostility. We were being cheated. We felt that the population was being cheated. We thought we gave great care, and had a great reputation for educating the best nurses in the country. And we just felt robbed of that. . . ."[108] At the PGH annual alumni reunion banquet held the Friday before to welcome the new graduates of the final class, alumni association president Florence Baker said, ". . . the spirit of Old Blockley will live on as long as there are still nurses who wear the double frill cap."[109] For all intents and purposes the graduation of the final class of PGH nurses became a requiem for PGH.

On June 17, 1977, 13 days before its scheduled closure, the last eight acute care patients were transferred to other facilities. Four hundred patients who would require nursing home care continued to be housed in one of the PGH buildings until the former Landis State Hospital was fully converted into its new incarnation as a nursing home. All ambulatory services had been transferred to either the city neighborhood health centers or one of five hospitals—Presbyterian, Graduate, Misericordia, Hahnemann, or St. Luke's—which had executed contracts with the city to provide care for the poor who formerly used PGH. Emergency care would be provided by the 30 hospitals closest to the patients needing urgent care.[110]

The end of an era—of William Osler and Alice Fisher—had come. The tradition of seeking excellence in the delivery of care, in concert with government as its agent, was past.

Notes

1. Executive Committee minutes, January 14, 1976. UPC 56.2, Box 3, University of Pennsylvania, PGH Archives.

2. UPC 52.6, Box 6, University of Pennsylvania, PGH Archives. In this meeting, Tina Weintraub also mentioned that a group of PGH medical staff was planning a visit to Baltimore City Hospital later that same month, where a similar program was enacted with success.

3. See correspondence to Patrick Storey from Tina Weintraub, January 26, 1976. UPC 52.6, Box 6, University of Pennsylvania, PGH Archives.

4. Hoag Levins, "PGH: Death by Neglect...Supply, Staff Shortages Killing Patients," *Philadelphia Daily News*, January 26, 1976, Polk private archives, Barbara Bates Center for Nursing History, University of Pennsylvania, clipping file.

5. Ibid.

6. Ibid.

7. Hoag Levins, "PGH: Shortage of Nurses Endanger Patients," *Philadelphia Daily News*, January 27, 1976.

8. Ibid.

9. Hoag Levins, "Nurse-Juggling Act Hid Shortage from HEW," *Philadelphia Daily News*, January 27, 1976.

10. Hoag Levins, "Inside PGH," *Philadelphia Daily News*, January 28, 1976.

11. Hoag Levins, "PGH Chairman Sells to His Own Hospital," *Philadelphia Daily News*, January 28, 1976.

12. Hoag Levins, "PGH Flunks PA Standard, Still Licensed," *Philadelphia Daily News*, January 29, 1976.

13. Hoag Levins, "Is PGH Doomed?" *Philadelphia Daily News*, January 30, 1976.

14. Ibid.

15. Hoag Levins, "Prosecution at PGH?" *Philadelphia Daily News*, January 31, 1976.

16. See the *Philadelphia Tribune* Archives at the Free Library of Philadelphia. Elaine Welles, "NAACP Asks to Place PGH Under Receivership," *Philadelphia Tribune*, January 31, 1976, p. 1; Elaine Welles, "NAACP Hits Filthy, Unsafe Conditions at Philadelphia General," *Philadelphia Tribune*, February 7, 1976.

17. Editorial by Gil Spencer, *Philadelphia Daily News*, February 3, 1976, Polk private archives, clipping file.

18. "42 Staff Doctors Demand Action at PGH," *Philadelphia Daily News*, February 3, 1976.

19. Chuck Stone, "PGH: The Making and Destroying of Niggers," *Philadelphia Daily News*, February 3, 1976.

20. Hoag Levins, "State Knew PGH Was Coming Up Short," *Philadelphia Daily News*, February 10, 1976.

21. Hoag Levins, "Watchdog Agency to Inspect PGH," *Philadelphia Daily News*, February 11, 1976.

22. The job freeze at PGH was ordered intermittently by the city administration as the PGH budget tightened, and City Council negotiations on the overall city budget continued without agreement.

23. PGH minutes, records and correspondence, February 6, 1976. UPC 56.2, Box 3, University of Pennsylvania, PGH Archives.

24. Ibid.

25. Special session minutes, February 9, 1976. UPC 56.2, Box 3, University of Pennsylvania, PGH Archives.

26. Executive Committee minutes, February 11, 1976. UPC 56.2, Box 3, University of Pennsylvania, PGH Archives.

27. Ibid.

28. Executive Committee minutes, February 16, 1976. UPC 56.2, Box 3, University of Pennsylvania, PGH Archives.

29. See oral history interview by author with Dr. Lewis Polk, Philadelphia, December 11, 2000.

30. See oral history interview by author with Stephanie Stachniewicz, Philadelphia, January 25, 2001, and February 15, 2001.

31. See the copy of the statement in the Polk private archives dated February 16, 1976.

32. In an interview by the author with Hillel Levinson, he mentioned that in addition to the demonstration, he was "burned in effigy" in the courtyard of City Hall, although the news reports reviewed did not mention this (Philadelphia, February 19, 2004).

33. "Decision on PGH Final, Mayor Says," *Philadelphia Bulletin*, February 18, 1976. The *Bulletin* Archives were retrieved from the *Bulletin* Morgue and are now in the Temple University Urban Archives.

34. John Gillespie, "Union Leaders Organize March to Protest PGH Closing Plan," *Philadelphia Bulletin*, February 18, 1976.

35. "Schwartz Seeks Parlay on PGH," *Philadelphia Bulletin*, 18 February 1976.

36. Letter to Mayor Rizzo from Chairman Perloff, dated February 18, 1976, and copied to all the members of the Board of Trustees, of which Dr. Polk was a member exofficio (Polk private archives).

37. Executive Committee minutes, February 18, 1976. UPC 56.2, Box 3, University of Pennsylvania, PGH Archives.

38. Ibid. Copy of statement in the Polk private archives. While it is not clear what the objections were, it is likely that they had to do with the quality of care, since the house staff was on record numerous times saying that they were not able to give good quality medical care due to the nursing shortage, the multiple missing supplies, and the delays in getting tests done and/or getting test results.

39. Executive Committee minutes, February 16, 1976. UPC 56.2, Box 3, University of Pennsylvania, PGH Archives.

40. Gunter David and John Dubois, "Meetings, Hearings Planned on PGH," *Philadelphia Bulletin*, February 20, 1976.

41. Hoag Levins, "Legislator Asks for PGH Probe," *Philadelphia Bulletin*, February 21, 1976.

42. David Cleary, "Ethel Allen Outlines Steps to Save PGH," *Philadelphia Bulletin*, February 22, 1976.

43. "Judge Overturns Ban on Rizzo's Decision to Close PGH," *Daily Pennsylvanian*, February 25, 1976.

44. Professor Sparer was also the author of an extensive report regarding the PGH closure. Edward V. Sparer, *Medical School Accountability in the Public Hospital: The University of Pennsylvania Medical School and the Philadelphia General Hospital* (Unpublished report, The Health Law Project, University of Pennsylvania, October 1974).

45. "Judge Ruling Allows Closing of PGH," *Philadelphia Bulletin*, February 24, 1976.

46. Ibid.

47. "Protest Crowd Chants Recall," *Philadelphia Bulletin*, February 25, 1976; "Marchers Protest PGH Closing Plan," February 26, 1976.

48. In an interview by author with Hillel Levinson, he stated that his greatest disappointment with the closure of PGH was that they were not able to figure out a way to keep the nursing school. Levinson described the PGH School of Nursing as superb and believed that the loss of the school was a blow to the city and the region (Philadelphia, February 19, 2004).

49. David Cleary, "PGH Plans Are 'Fluid,' Health Council Told," *Philadelphia Bulletin*, February 26, 1976.

50. Gunter David, "3 Councilmen Urge Big Meeting on PGH," *Philadelphia Bulletin*, February 27, 1976.

51. Gunter David, "Protesters Join Forces to Blitz City Hall," *Philadelphia Bulletin*, March 12, 1976.

52. This analysis of Schwartz, and City Council's likely action, was included in "The PGH Battle," *Philadelphia Inquirer*, March 1, 1976.

53. See oral history interviews by author with Ernest Zeger (Carlisle, PA, June 22, 2003) and Stephanie Stachniewicz (Philadelphia, January 25, 2001, and February 15, 2001). Zeger stated that when he first became aware of the plans for the closure, he doubted it would really occur. Stachniewicz was not at all sure how to proceed with managing the issues surrounding the nursing school, and whether or not that might be a wedge to prevent the closure.

54. David Cleary, "PGH 'Inflates' Patient Lists, Polk Admits," *Philadelphia Bulletin*, March 18, 1976.

55. Ibid. The miscalculations were tied to counting the same patients as many as three or four times as they moved from one clinic to another within the system, and the fact that many of the inpatients were not true acute care patients, but rather custodial care patients who didn't "belong in anyone's hospital" because they could not get nursing home beds.

56. PGH Medical Staff Cabinet minutes, March 4, 1986. UPC 56.2, Box 3, University of Pennsylvania, PGH Archives.

57. Ibid.

58. PGH Medical Staff Cabinet minutes, April 1, 1976. UPC 56.2, Box 3, University of Pennsylvania, PGH Archives.

59. See transcript of oral history interview by author with Ernest Zeger (Carlisle, PA, June 22, 2003).

60. Executive Committee minutes, April 14, 1976. UPC 56.2, Box 3, University of Pennsylvania, PGH Archives.

61. PGH Medical Staff Cabinet minutes, March 4, 1986. UPC 56.2, Box 3, University of Pennsylvania, PGH Archives. In addition see Donald Drake, "While Awaiting a Plan for PGH, Some Speculation," *Philadelphia Inquirer*, March 21, 1976. This description of patients is also consistent with the oral history interview by the author with PGH student nurse Eileen Kelly (Philadelphia, July 29, 2003), who describes the diagnosis of "dispo" on many patient charts.

62. Drake, ibid.

63. Ibid.

64. "5 On Council Hit Lack of Data on PGH," *Philadelphia Bulletin*, April 20, 1976.

65. Ibid. Two days later, The *Bulletin* released a poll that indicated the public was against the PGH closure. In the poll, 500 city residents were asked if they were opposed to closing the hospital. Fifty-seven percent said they were against it, 19 percent said it made no difference to them, 16 percent thought it was a good idea, and 8 percent had expressed no concern.

66. Letter dated April 28, 1976, Polk private archives. The report referenced in the letter is attached.

67. Ibid.

68. Ibid. See the untitled report attached to the correspondence from Levinson to Schwartz. Also see "City Striving to Reach Pact on PGH patients," *Philadelphia Bulletin*, April 29, 1976.

69. Untitled report attached to the correspondence from Levinson to Schwartz, 2-3, Polk private archives.

70. Ibid., 5-6. The report also includes a map with the new district health centers identified, such that the geographical accessibility for city-wide services is highlighted, as compared to the less-accessible PGH (Appendix G).

71. Ibid., 6.

72. Ibid., 7.

73. Ibid., 7-8.

74. "Phila to Transfer 86 When Laundry Sold," *Philadelphia Bulletin*, April 30, 1976.

75. "Hospitals Ease Off on PGH," *Philadelphia Bulletin*, May 2, 1976.

76. "Hospitals Ask for More City Aid," *Philadelphia Bulletin*, May 3, 1976.

77. Executive Committee minutes, April 14, 1976. UPC 56.2, Box 3, University of Pennsylvania, PGH Archives.

78. Ibid.

79. See "Many PGH Doctors, Nurses Are Leaving," *Philadephia Bulletin*, May 5, 1976; "March to Protest Closing of PGH," *Philadelphia Bulletin*, May 11, 1976.

80. "PGH: The City Pulled the Plug," *Philadelphia Daily News*, May 13, 1976; "City Poor: PGH Crisis Pawns," *Philadelphia Daily News*, May 14, 1976.

81. "Hearse Leads March to Protest PGH Closing," *Philadelphia Bulletin*, May 23, 1976.

82. Executive Committee minutes, June 9, 1976. UPC 56.2, Box 3, University of Pennsylvania, PGH Archives.

83. Ibid. It is also interesting to note that in this same meeting the committee discussed the PGH bicentennial. They saw this event as an opportunity to memorialize the significant historical role PGH had played in the advent of medicine and nursing in the city and the nation. The committee planned to solicit and appropriate funds for the project using the content of the Osler Memorial Museum as the core of the exhibit. Here the committee appeared to be mindful of the emerging fact that PGH was passing, on their watch, into historical memory.

84. "PGH Plan Is Still Being Planned," *Philadelphia Daily News*, July 7, 1976; "PGH Closing Costs," *Philadelphia Daily News*, June 14, 1976.

85. "Court OKs End of PGH," *Philadelphia Bulletin*, August 13, 1976.

86. Ibid.

87. "Maternity Service at PGH Closed," *Philadelphia Bulletin*, September 30, 1976.

88. "PGH Outpatient Services to Be Moved to Centers," *Philadelphia Bulletin*, September 1, 1976.

89. Executive Committee minutes, September 8, 1976. UPC 56.2, Box 3, University of Pennsylvania, PGH Archives.

90. "Chaplain Won't Give Up Until the Doors Are Shut," *Philadelphia Bulletin*, October 10, 1976.

91. "Issues in PGH March," *Philadelphia Bulletin*, February 25, 1976. Also see transcript of oral history interview by author with Barry Savitz (Philadelphia, July 26, 2000) that confirms these approximate numbers and patient classifications.

92. Dr. Tom Storey, medical director of PGH is quoted in *Philadelphia Bulletin*, February 20, 1976, 4.

93. See oral history interview by author with Barry Savitz (Philadelphia, July 26, 2000).

94. Philadelphia Department of Public Health, *Comments and Analysis of the Hospital Survey Committee Report on Philadelphia General Hospital of May 28, 1972* (Philadelphia, 1972, Polk private archives).

95. See the report summary in Hospital Survey Committee, *Report and Recommendations of the Hospital Survey Committee with Respect to Alternatives for the Provision of Medical Care Now Rendered to the Citizens of Philadelphia at Philadelphia General Hospital* (Philadelphia, 1972, Polk private archives).

96. Ibid.

97. "Rizzo Reaffirms Private Hospitals Will Care for Poor," *Philadelphia Bulletin*, October 20, 1976. Also, in Executive Committee minutes of October 13, Dr. Gray (for Ambulatory Services) reported that the plan for enrolling patients in the family practice program in the District #2 Health Center seemed to be "progressing fairly well." Executive Committee minutes, October 13, 1976. UPC 56.2, Box 3, University of Pennsylvania, PGH Archives.

98. "Problems with the PGH Problem," *Philadelphia Inquirer*, December 14, 1976.

99. Executive Committee minutes, November 10, 1976. UPC 56.2, Box 3, University of Pennsylvania, PGH Archives.

100. Executive Committee minutes, January 12, 1977. UPC 56.2, Box 3, University of Pennsylvania, PGH Archives. In this archive, see the comments on Stephanie Stachniewicz under psychiatry regarding the prospects for getting nurses. Also see that "Mr. Devlin seems to be in favor of a museum on the grounds," regarding the disposition of PGH collections." Most importantly, these minutes detail the

plans for the Health Department to transition the PGH ambulatory patients into their system. According to Barry Savitz who was charged with achieving as seamless a transition as possible, all patients were able to keep their own physician when they got their new "medical home" in the city clinics. See the Savitz oral history interview for more details on the patient transition.

101. Executive Committee minutes, February 8, 1977. UPC 56.2, Box 3, University of Pennsylvania, PGH Archives.

102. Ibid.

103. Executive Committee minutes, April 9, 1977. UPC 56.2, Box 3, University of Pennsylvania, PGH Archives.

104. Executive Committee minutes, May 11, 1977. UPC 56.2, Box 3, University of Pennsylvania, PGH Archives.

105. Ibid. Dr. Heaton also announced in this final meeting that awards would be given to the members of the Executive Committee and the chairmen of standing committees, which would be fashioned from wood from the old PGH amphitheater and bricks from the pathology building.

106. Ibid.

107. See "City Finds Ways to Soften Loss of PGH," *Philadelphia Inquirer*, 27 March 1977; "The PGH Shutdown Proceeds," *Philadelphia Daily News*, April 14, 1977; "19 Hospitals to Aid Patients," *Philadelphia Bulletin*, April 30, 1977; "When PGH Closes, Regulars Will Lose," *Philadelphia Bulletin*, May 2, 1977; "Future for PGH Male Nurse: City Offers Him Janitor Job," *Philadelphia Bulletin*, May 29, 1977.

108. See transcript of oral history interview by author with Eileen Kelly (Philadelphia, July 29, 2003).

109. "Old Blockley Nurses: Pride, Tradition Live On in the Double Frill Cap," *Philadelphia Bulletin*, May 19, 1977.

110. "Last Patients Transferred from PGH," *Philadelphia Bulletin*, June 18, 1977.

6

PGH: The Decision and the Aftermath

One of the baffling things about life is that the purpose of institutions may be ideal, while their administration, dependent upon the faults and weaknesses of human beings, may be bad.

Mary Barnett Gibson[1]

The Decision

I was brought in by Rizzo several times. . . It wasn't like he was walking blindly into this thing. . . He knew the anti-Rizzo forces were looking for an issue, and this was the perfect issue for them because it involved the closing of a hospital that to him at the time that he was going to get his head handed to him on this issue, even though it was the right decision. Everybody agreed it was the right decision. And he said, 'The only thing I care about is making the right decision. I have spent my entire life dealing with controversial things. I have no problem with that.' That was what happened. . . .

We never did any polling [on the decision to close the hospital]. He was never interested in that. I would just say, 'Let me poll the issues,' and he would say, "I don't give a shit what people think. I want to do what is right."

Excerpt from an oral history interview with
Martin "Marty" Weinberg, former City Solicitor
and political advisor to Mayor Frank Rizzo.[2]

91

When we first started reviewing this, he [Mayor Rizzo] was absolute-
ly opposed to closing PGH. Again, I think it was an emotional thing
for him. He remembers the days he went in there as a cop and was
treated very well. He started at the point all the way on one side,
which was "Over my dead body you're going to close PGH". . . . Once
he realized that it was the right decision, come hell or high water, we
were going to go ahead and do it. Marty was giving him the right
decision politically [not to close it], there's no question about it. . .
[but] he was not going to knuckle under to the abuse he was going
to take in order to make the right decision.

> Excerpt from an oral history interview with
> Hillel Levinson, Managing Director of the City of
> Philadelphia under Mayor Frank Rizzo.[3]

When Frank Rizzo and his cabinet came into office in January
1972, they inherited a Philadelphia General Hospital that had a long,
well-documented history of administrative problems coupled with an
increasingly complex fiscal and bureaucratic environment. According to Levinson, Mayor Rizzo began his administration with a favorable disposition toward PGH, influenced by his history as a Philadelphia police officer, and that of his brother Joe Rizzo as a fireman who
would later be Fire Commissioner. The sense that they had upon taking office was that PGH had some problems. ". . . Let's see if we can
figure out a way to make this work. But four years into the administration, maybe even earlier than that, it became obvious that there
was just no way to make this thing work. . . ."[4]

In a meeting with Levinson in late January of 1976,[5] Rizzo told
him that the decision had been made and asked him to make the
announcement. Levinson knew there would be a significant public
reaction. He was right. In the days and months that followed, Levinson was stalked and his home picketed. He was burned in effigy in
the City Hall courtyard, and received death threats. It was the first
time in his city service that he was assigned a police bodyguard and
the first time he felt that one was actually needed.[6]

The reaction to the closure by certain public groups became the
centerpiece in a larger political context. At the same time the PGH
decision was made, a group of Rizzo supporters, with his approval,[7]
began to advance a change in the City Charter to permit the mayor
to serve more than two terms. The Charter change movement
became a political flashpoint in the city, and opponents used the

PGH closure to further energize the anti-Charter change forces. These high emotions contributed mightily to a climate of unrest. The closure of the hospital was swept into the political maelstrom, making it more difficult to separate substance from politics.

Intractable Matters in Public Policy

In October 1974, University of Pennsylvania professor Edward Sparer, under the auspices of the Health Law Project, issued a controversial report evaluating the complex relationship between the university and PGH.[8] In the report, Sparer provided an exhaustive analysis of the inherent conflicts associated with the contracting agreements between the city, on behalf of PGH, and the university, and, by extension, the other contracting medical schools. In his conclusions, Sparer argued that there should be "informed public debate," and that the goal of the report was to generate that debate and enable a "public decision-making process conducted with maximum information including information on the entrepreneurial interests and needs of the medical school groups."[9] Sparer made several recommendations for changes to the affiliation contract, quality of care standards, and the quality review board, in which expanded capacity could permit more independence. The report offered many other detailed recommendations, including those for salaries and operating principles. But what is most intriguing about the report are the factors not analyzed and considered.

While Sparer made "governance" recommendations, he never considered the possibility that PGH could become an entity separate from the city and seek nonprofit status, a process many public hospitals were actively pursuing. In addition, Sparer failed to address the issue of capital financing. The October report did not note, discuss, or review the creation of the Philadelphia Hospital Authority which occurred in January 1974, ten months before Sparer issued his study findings,[10] nor the public hearings conducted on the creation of the Authority held the year before.[11] The study, which alluded to the need for upgrading the facilities, did not fully consider all the data available at the time. This limitation in the study subverted the capacity to achieve the investigator's stated goal of "public discussion with maximum available information."[12]

However, Sparer's study does provide us with important insights into the complexities of interorganizational relationships.

While his recommendations might be useful in a functioning organization, at the stage in which this study was conducted there were too
many complexities converging into different public policy conclusions.[13] The recommendations are telling in that they point out, in
extensive operational minutiae, the improbability of their application.[14]

Once the closure was announced, Sparer's report served as a
public policy rallying cry by those opposed to the PGH closing. Dr.
Walter Lear, a deputy commissioner in the Department of Public
Health, used Sparer's report, in part, as the basis for his opposition
to the closing. Lear was an active member of Americans for Democratic Action (ADA), which became one of the principal opposition
groups to the Rizzo administration and the PGH closing.[15] Sparer
also served as part of the legal team assembled by attorney and former mayoral candidate Charles Bowser, who sued the city to prevent
the closure. In his findings in the report, Sparer directly cited the city
government as having "abdicated its role."[16]

The Role of City Government
and the "Strong Mayor" Model

In fact, city government had not abdicated its role but had fulfilled it
as defined by the arrangement and allocation of political power,
reaching back to the Act of Consolidation of 1854. The act provided
for a measure of political reform and significant structural change by
redefining city boundaries, thereby increasing the significance and
power of the mayor. This was soon followed by another iteration of
reform, including the Charter change of 1885 and the Bullit Bill in
1887. These legislative initiatives provided for further delineation of
responsibility, more of which was vested in the mayor.[17] They also
decreased the power of City Council. Other changes to the structure
of City Council and department heads emerged over time.[18] But the
"strong mayor" form of government gave Frank Rizzo, and his
appointees, a wide-ranging scope of decision-making and policy
implementation power. That Mayor Rizzo, and his administration,
decided and acted to close PGH was completely consistent with the
design and expectations of the City Charter.

The Board of PGH, while an independent body, drew all of its
appointments, including the chairman, from the mayor, under whose
aegis they served.[19] The nature of the relationships appointees have

to the appointing authority (in this case the mayor) is one of dynamic tension. Sometimes the expectations of each may not be in concert. The appointees may expect to be the actual decision-makers, or at least to be consulted on major matters. The appointing authority may or may not share that paradigm of the relationship. In the case of PGH, when the announcement of the closure was made, Earl Perloff, the chairman of the PGH board appointed by Mayor Rizzo, resigned. In the end, the "strong mayor" form of government supersedes any expectations.

In a related structural matter, the Department of Public Health was the operating department within city government charged with oversight of PGH. The Health Commissioner also served on the Board of Trustees of PGH.[20] Further, the Managing Director's office had assigned a deputy managing director, Tina Weintraub, to oversee the day-to-day issues of PGH. Again, all of the executive level staff and board appointees were empowered in their roles by the mayor, who was the appointing authority in each and every instance. This clearly reflects the spirit and the structure of the "strong mayor" form of government, which permitted Mayor Rizzo the political and governmental latitude to effect the closure.

The Issue of Race and the PGH Closure

The issue of race was both a flashpoint and a context for many aspects of the closure. Race played a central role in the perception of PGH, in that a preponderance of its patient population was African American and poor, in terms of the care delivered within the institution, and in the attitude of the administration, especially the mayor, with regard to his disposition toward African-American Philadelphians.[21] A large portion of the city union workforce that would be eliminated by the closure of PGH was African American.[22] Multiple allegations were made that Mayor Frank Rizzo was racist, and that he was closing a hospital that was regarded as the community property of non-Caucasian citizens of the city. It was also alleged that Rizzo "starved" the hospital because he was not concerned about the minority community or the care they received.[23] While the notion of Rizzo as a racist fit nicely into the contemporary political paradigm, was useful for the anti-Rizzo forces within the city, and offered a simple explanation for the closure of PGH, other factors in administra-

tive behavior and in Rizzo's official acts do not permit such a sim-
plistic conclusion.[24]

The amount of planning and reorganization that went into the
transition of the closure and the associated expenses suggest that the
implementation of the decision, while difficult and politically unpop-
ular, was thoughtful, deliberative, and for the most part, well-execut-
ed.[25] A new nursing home that maximized the county's reimbursement stream was developed. All PGH patients were transitioned into
the nursing home or into an ambulatory care setting that was more
geographically convenient and allowed them to keep their primary
care physicians.[26] This act of continuity in health care delivery, a
clear advantage for quality patient care, would be no longer feasible
in contemporary health care contexts.

Ironically, the PGH closure, while adding fuel to the "Recall
Rizzo" effort, contributed significantly to the desegregation of the
Philadelphia hospital network. With PGH closed, the nonprofit hospitals accepted patients regardless of race with more alacrity in order
to receive Medicare/Medicaid reimbursements, which included
strong measures preventing segregation in health care delivery. In an
earlier and important action, the Equal Employment Opportuny
Commission (EEOC) launched an effort to integrate African-American physicians into positions in more Philadelphia hospitals. The
aggressive effort undertaken in Philadelphia through the 1960's and
'70's, headed by Congressman Robert N.C. Nix and social scientist
Sadie Mosell-Alexander, led to a dramatic rise in the number of
African-American physicians serving in leadership and patient care
roles. This integration increased the probability that African-American patients would go to a hospital traditionally used by white
Philadelphians, since physicians of their own race could care for
them.[27] One of the reasons that many African Americans sought care
at PGH was the fact that PGH, unlike many other hospitals, established a clear nondiscrimination policy as part of a City Charter
change in 1953. The new reimbursement structure and the new
EEOC oversight pushed the other city hospitals toward equitable and
nondiscriminatory access.[28]

Notes

1. Mary Barnett Gibson, born in 1877, was a factory personnel manager, an economist, and an educator. Mary Barnett Gibson, "What's Past Is Prologue," in *The Columbia World of Quotations* (New York: Columbia University Press, 1996), chapter 27, no. 24947.

2. See oral history interview by author with Martin Weinberg, Philadelphia, July 28, 2003. The quote reflects Weinberg's recollection of what Mayor Rizzo said to him in this meeting.

3. See oral history interview by author with Hillel Levinson, Philadelphia, February 19, 2004.

4. Ibid.

5. Levinson remembers this meeting as occurring sometime shortly after the mayor was inaugurated for a second term, which by City Charter is required to take place on the first Tuesday of the New Year after the November election.

6. See oral history interview by author with Hillel Levinson, Philadelphia, February 19, 2004.

7. The Charter change was counter to Weinberg's political advice to Rizzo. See the Weinberg oral history interview on the subject of the city Charter change.

8. Edward V. Sparer, *Medical School Accountability in the Public Hospital: The University of Pennsylvania Medical School and the Philadelphia General Hospital* (Unpublished report, The Heath Law Project, University of Pennsylvania, October 1974), in the Polk private archives. Professor Sparer joined the faculty of PENN's law school in 1969, and at that time he established the Health Law Project. The Health Law Project operated under the aegis of the law school for more than a decade, providing legal assistance in many health care-related legal challenges, of which the PGH issue was one. Eventually, the Health Law Project became the Pennsylvania Health Law Project, which is now located on Cherry Street in Philadelphia. It sponsors the Sparer Public Interest Fellowship, named for the late professor.

9. Ibid., 107-108.

10. See the history of the Philadelphia Hospital Authority, discussed in Chapter 4.

11. Sparer.

12. Ibid., 107.

13. John W. Kingdon, *Agendas, Alternatives, and Public Policies*, 2nd ed. (New York: Longman, 2003).

14. See Sparer's conclusions; Sparer, 93-116.

15. See oral history interview by author with Dr. Walter Lear, Philadelphia, July 30, 2003, and his writings on the subject of the PGH closing, in Lear private archives, Institute of Social Medicine and Community Health, Philadelphia.

16. Sparer, 2.

17. John Welsh Croskey, *History of Blockley* (Philadelphia: F. A. Davis, 1929), 71-72.

18. For a fulsome review of the changes in city government that resulted in the "strong mayor" form of government, see Pennsylvania Economy League, *Philadelphia Government*, 6th ed. (Philadelphia, 1963).

19. See the oral history interview by author with former Health Commissioner Lewis Polk (Philadelphia, December 11, 2000), who describes his role on the PGH Board of Trustees. Polk also said that even though he was not responsible for the PGH closure decision, which came from Mayor Rizzo through Managing Director Hillel Levinson, he faced great reaction from friends, family, and colleagues, who felt he should have resigned when the decision was made.

20. Ibid.

21. See Weinberg, oral history interview.

22. Ibid.

23. See Lear, oral history interview.

24. Other observations regarding Frank Rizzo, in the context of race, merit consideration and discussion. Many of Rizzo's opponents believed that he was a racist who would be inclined to close PGH. His supporters categorically deny both allegations. According to Hillel Levinson (oral history interview by author, Philadelphia, February 19, 2004), "Frank was not a racist. That just wasn't true...he had good experiences with PGH as a cop...when we came into office, we thought that it [PGH] was something that had problems, and we would figure out a way to fix it." Lieutenant Anthony Fulwood (oral history interview by author, Philadelphia, July 23, 2003), one of the first African-American police officers assigned by Mayor Rizzo to an elite security unit, continues to assert that Frank Rizzo was not a racist. "You know, he was a giver to the underdog. He didn't care if you were white or black or anything. If you needed help, he will be there for you. He didn't want to see anyone taken advantage of, no matter what color you are," said Fulwood, who reminisced about Frank Rizzo as a fair man who was misunderstood. "I worked for the man for years, and I've seen him at his weakest and most vulnerable times, and he never showed any signs of racism. In fact, he had more black friends than white friends. If you go to his house on Saturday morning, everybody is up at his house sitting around." Other people connected to Mayor Rizzo support Fulwood's contention. Joe Rizzo, who served as Fire Commissioner in his brother's administration, recalls that when Frank Rizzo was a captain in the 19th police district, he was the first captain to integrate police cars, assigning one Caucasian officer and one African-American officer to sector patrol cars. Joe Rizzo (oral history interview by author, Philadelphia, June 25, 2003) believed that "the higher ranks in the police department were a little upset with what he did [integrating police officer patrols]." In the larger political context, the label "racist" was a useful political tool. Because Rizzo was large, gruff, ethnic, and not college-educated, he was, in many ways, ideally situated to be characterized, even caricatured, as a racist. However, there are other facts about Rizzo that bear additional weight in the public perception. Having lost his mother to an early death and suffering physical abuse as an adolescent, Frank Rizzo was an angry man (see oral history interview with Hillel Levinson). That anger found expression in a lack of tolerance for complexity and a willingness and propensity to react in fury. In any context in which race might play a role, this could easily translate into a perception of racism. In fact, it was classism. Frank Rizzo was comfortable with poor and working-class people of all races but he was not at all comfortable with the city elite— the college-educated, newspaper-writing, and liberal wing of the Democratic Party. The best way to discredit Rizzo politically was to call him a racist. Rizzo reacted to that charge with the anger that had become part of his legend. This cyclic engagement produced a divided city, in what came to be regarded by members of Americans for Democratic Action as "Free Philadelphia" and "Rizzo Philadelphia." See the oral history interview by the author with Lenora Berson, an active member of the ADA and one of the key advocates for the recall of Frank

Rizzo (Philadelphia, January 15, 2001). This was, in part, a driving factor in the "Recall Rizzo" movement and in the defeat of the Charter change that would have permitted the mayor to be reelected to more than two terms. Also see the oral history interview with Weinberg, and S.A. Paolantonio, *Frank Rizzo: The Last Big Man in Big City America* (Philadelphia: Camino Books, 1993), chapters 11 and 13.

25. See the oral history interviews with Weinberg, Polk (Philadelphia, December 11, 2000), Levinson, and Stachniewicz (Philadelphia, January 25, 2001, and February 15, 2001). Also see the previously cited newspaper articles in chapter 5 from the *Philadelphia Daily News* and the *Philadelphia Inquirer* from 1977. During this part of the transition, the costs associated with the transfer of contract services and the development and implementation of the extensive new network of family medical practice service within the Department of Public Health were very substantial. Also see the oral history interview by the author with Barry Savitz (Philadelphia, July 26, 2000), which discusses the relocation of all the PGH patients so that they maintained their primary care physicians. This accomplishment in continuity of care is something that likely could not be achieved in contemporary health care delivery.

26. Ibid. Barry Savitz was a medical center director placed in charge of the transition of patients into these new settings.

27. David McBride, *Integrating the City of Medicine: Blacks in Philadelphia Health Care 1910-1965* (Philadelphia: Temple University Press, 1989), 196-198.

28. Ibid., 171.

7

Analysis, Discussion, and Final Thoughts

There are many challenges in unraveling the decision to close Philadelphia General Hospital. The process of sorting and assigning value to the facts, the motivations, the political machinations, and the context from rumors, suppositions, and assumptions is a difficult analytic task and a somewhat intuitive challenge faced by all historians. Doing so in a public policy context, and in such a highly charged political environment, heightens the difficulty. The objective data clearly point toward collapse of the institution.

Based on a reexamination and analysis of the Alpha Center study (described in Chapter 3) from the perspective of PGH, seven of the eight internal factors and four of the six external factors militated against the survival of PGH.

The Alpha Center Study Revisited

The Financial Condition of the Hospital
At the time the closure announcement was made, PGH had been beset by multiple financial difficulties. Ongoing struggles between the hospital management, the participating medical schools, the city administration, and the City Council were well known and documented in the public record and within the institutions. Contracts for services

were often delayed pending appropriations. Interinstitutional turf battles over what got funded, and by whom, were standard practice. Moreover, the capacity to resolve these issues was often elusive.[1]

Management and Administrative Problems Associated with Government Bureaucracy

The complex arrangements and relationships that PGH constructed and sought to maintain with its constituent members were an ongoing source of struggle. Over the course of more than 30 years, multiple blue-ribbon panels and commissions were charged with addressing the problems, consistently revealing the complexity of the bureaucracy. Civil service rules were often cited as a hiring problem since the rules were inconsistent with the emerging practices of local nonprofit hospitals. Conflicts with medical schools over control, responsibilities, and resources, and the resulting negotiations that produced agreements buckled the best of collegial intentions. Often the conflict between the city government and the medical schools over contract issues dragged on so far into the fiscal year that by the time one annual contract battle ended, another one ensued.[2]

Condition of the Physical Plant and Equipment

The physical plant of PGH, at the time of the closure decision, was clearly a major factor in its demise. A study by Medicon, authorized by the Department of Public Health, clearly stated that the PGH "physical plant was found to be totally obsolete, and expensive to operate."[3] The city expressed concern over the cost of building a new facility. In addition, at the time of the closure, the University of Pennsylvania Hospital was adjacent to the PGH site, and there were already discussions of moving the Children's Hospital of Philadelphia (CHOP) to a new site, also adjacent to PGH. These well-appointed, well-funded, and modern facilities were encroaching upon the role that PGH had historically occupied.

The Ability to Raise Capital

At the time of the PGH closure, Philadelphia's nonprofit hospitals were at the height of a capitalized remodernization boom. The establishment of the Philadelphia Hospital Authority in January 1974 had positioned it to acquire access to low-cost capital via tax-exempt financing. Philanthropic funds, although useful for leverage and always valuable, were not sufficient to the task and traditional bank financing was cost-prohibitive. These new tax-exempt bonds were critical since Hill-Burton funds, which supplied the first postwar wave of financing for hospital expansion, had dried up. The non-profit bonds issued by the authority would not affect the city's bond rating since they were obligated by only the nonprofits themselves. With many municipalities facing significant financial distress, the status of the city's bond rating was of central importance to the administration and to other elected officials. What this meant, functionally, was that since PGH was a city-owned public entity, the hospital was in a disadvantaged position to acquire access to these funds.[4] To do so would require the city to obligate future revenues, which, based on the previous fiscal practices and performance of PGH, would clearly imperil the fiscal health of the city writ large. Based on the City Council hearings, in which the creation of the Philadelphia Hospital Authority was considered and later created, a primary objective for the Rizzo administration was to limit fiscal liability. In doing so, the administration sought to protect the integrity of the city's fiscal stability. It offset this interest by creating access for the nonprofit hospitals to tax-exempt capital with the creation of the Hospital Authority, including a series of provisos and contracts that brought the nonprofits toward a higher level of commitment to the poor, the aged, and other categorical groups that had previously been PGH constituencies.

The Ability to Attract Adequate and Competent Staff
PGH had a well-documented problem with recruiting and retaining nurses.[5] Rumors that the hospital would close, and the mandatory civil service system, impinged on the hospital's ability to attract and retain nurses, as well as physicians. Although PGH had its own nursing school and kept a portion of its graduates, this still was not enough. As the hospital declined, more physicians exited. This further complicated the need to sustain the contractual relationships with the medical schools

The Ability to Attract Patients
PGH had a few defined patient constituencies: police and firemen, who were required, except in cases of extreme emergency, to be cared for at the city hospital; and the poor, often African-American, who

were the traditional patients of PGH, dating back to its early incarnation as an almshouse. But patients that now had either employer-
based insurance or Medicare/Medicaid had an increasing number of
options around the city. Over time this became an increasing problem. With the emerging dominance of nonprofit hospitals and PGH's
declining public reputation, patients began to seek their care in other
locations.[6] In years leading up to the PGH closure, the patients who
increasingly resided in PGH beds were "disposition cases," meaning
they had nowhere else to go upon discharge.

The Effects of the Teaching Programs on the Operation of the Hospital

PGH's teaching programs were world-renowned for many decades.[7]
In the years preceding the closure, conflict escalated among the participating medical schools. The authorized structure called for the
medical schools, by contractual relationship, to manage and deliver
the medical care in the hospital. The main components were the "A"
Division, for which the University of Pennsylvania had principal
responsibility. PENN later entered into a contract with Jefferson
Medical College to provide service, but retained overall control. Similarly, in Division "B," Temple University Medical School had overall
responsibility, and later contracted with both the Women's' Medical
College of Pennsylvania and Hahnemann Medical School to share
the provision of services. Ongoing battles over contracts, allocated
resources, and division of available disbursements threatened these
collegial agreements. Eventually, the contracts collapsed under the
weight of the conflict.[8]

The Attitude of the Board and/or Government Officials Toward the Hospital

Over the years, multiple blue-ribbon panels sought to address the
longstanding problems of PGH. The 1970 report from Mayor Tate's
Committee on Municipal Hospital Services described PGH as public
policy's first concern, stating, "Despite the progress from a tighter
organization of the Philadelphia Department of Public Health, one
institution defied the science of public administration. That was the
PGH. And to this day, it continues to confound policy-makers in their
attempt to reorganize it, or make it a rational part of the health care
system."[9] So frustrated was Mayor Tate with the systematic intransi-

gence that he sought the assistance of the University of Pennsylvania to take over PGH.[10]

The Attitude of the Citizenry Toward the Facility

At the time the closure was announced, PGH was widely regarded as a failing institution by the external world. The extensive, negative publicity generated by a series of exposé-type articles by Hoag Levinson at the *Philadelphia Daily News* framed the public view of the hospital. Horror stories of poor medical and patient care abounded. Public conflict among the leading contractual medical institutions contributed to a sense that the hospital was in a state of disarray. This contrasted significantly with the internal view of staff, who believed that the public reports were sensationalized and were inconsistent with the realities of what they believed to be the case: that PGH provided excellent patient care despite its obsolete physical plant.[11]

The Fiscal Condition of the County or Municipality

The City of Philadelphia, like many other urban areas, was facing significant federal cutbacks. In addition, public employee contracts that had been negotiated in the previous administration now had to be put into effect, which required a major tax increase. Soon after Mayor Rizzo was reelected, a significant wage tax hike was put into effect, enraging the voters who reelected him. Meanwhile, New York City, which had one of the most expansive public hospital systems of any city, was facing bankruptcy. The potential fiscal collapse of New York was a clarion call to all cities, whose elected leadership took notice. There was a sense that cities, as a general matter, were facing increasing fiscal instability. That necessitated a reconsideration of major expenditures. PGH, by virtue of its sheer size and financial needs, was at the top of that list. These issues framed the thinking of elected officials and citizens who were being asked to pay more in local taxes without the guarantee that additional revenues would be enough.[12]

The Attitude of Private Community Clinics

A group of health care activists led by Dr. Walter Lear, then Deputy Health Commissioner, sought to organize the local medical society, the unions, Americans for Democratic Action, and other constituencies to prevent the PGH closure, which included a failed lawsuit to that end.[13] Most other key providers in the Philadelphia health care community were ambivalent about the closure. Lear asserted that this ambivalence was rooted in self-serving behavior, since the new community hospitals were now competing with the old, obsolete PGH to deliver care to the Medicare and Medicaid populations of patients, who now enjoyed reimbursable coverage for delivered care.

The Extent to Which the Hospital Is a Source of Employment for Inner City Residents

This was a key factor and a key strategy of the Rizzo administration's need to politically neutralize the most important constituency of the "Keep PGH" movement—1199C. This was the largest union of PGH employees, numbering 5,000 city-wide. Most were minority and blue-collar workers. In order to blunt the criticism that Rizzo faced, he announced that no layoffs from the closure would occur. All PGH employees would be given new positions within city government. This important concession by the Rizzo administration was regarded as the single biggest factor in slowing the momentum of the anti-closure forces.[14]

The Overall Supply of Hospital Beds in the Community

In the late 1960's, only a few years after the passage of Medicare and Medicaid, Philadelphia had 6.5 beds per 1000 population. The national standard at that time was 2.5 beds per 1000 population. The occupancy rate was about 78.5 percent.[15] In 1971, there were 13,150 available acute care beds city-wide, of which 44 percent (or 5,839) did not conform to the standards established by the U.S. Public Health Service.[16] At the time that the PGH closure was announced, the number of conforming hospital beds was increasing in nonprofit hospitals, directly related to the establishment of the Philadelphia Hospital Authority, spurring reinvestment in hospital modernization.

The Demographic and Health Status Characteristics of the County or Municipality

Since many of the previously uninsured were now covered by Medicare or Medicaid, the demographics of the patient population at PGH in the waning years changed. Many of the patients were chronic in nature, and not exhibiting the characteristics of what was then considered "good medical material," meaning interesting, challenging cases. Most of the preferred acute patients were migrating into other, better-equipped teaching hospitals.[17]

Lens of Public Policy

Public policy experts and public administration scholars differ in their views on the closure of large-scale institutions. An argument can be made that the closure of PGH was a clash of cultures: multiple bureaucratic views colliding with the emerging entrepreneurship embodied by the medical schools and their affiliated hospitals. The bureaucratic culture[18] is hallmarked by a variety of specific organizational traits that resulted from multiple theories about capacities and functions of bureaucracies. Some bureaucratic theorists might ascribe "organizational psychology" as the most relevant of the applicable theories since it asserts the notion that an institution develops a "psyche." The emerging dynamic seeks to incorporate its human membership into the larger organism, such that they become subcomponents of the organization (PGH). That PGH possessed this organizational psyche and was unable to incorporate the other human/organizational components may explain, from that theoretical framework, why PGH's bureaucracy failed.[19]

One of the most fascinating phenomena of PGH, which supports the notion of institutional psyche, is the continuing PGH reunion. Held every year in the first week of May, former members of the PGH community gather to commemorate the tradition of PGH. At an annual dinner reception, former PGH executives, nurses, physicians, staff, patients, and families reminisce and enjoy the fellowship of their storied institution. The fact that these reunions still occur, more than 25 years after the closing, speaks volumes about the depth of feeling still held by PGH loyalists, and the shared identity that still resides within this unique group.

Another public policy lens through which one can view the PGH closure requires the reconciliation of the notions of randomness and rationality in applied public policy.[20] Theorists of this paradigm argue that separate "streams" of phenomena "couple" or converge around a problem. The convergence, or coupling, is chaotic and unpredictable, resulting in "organized anarchy." The three streams that converge include the problems and potential solutions that are recognized and refined into policy proposals and politics. The fluidity with which these phenomena converge creates a chaotic process. The resulting chaos creates "windows of opportunity" that are then exploited by the major actors in the policy-setting arena, or "policy entrepreneurs." Often, some type of "focusing event" drives the problem to the top of the policy agenda and toward a policy resolution.

Clearly in the PGH closure, all of these factors were at work over a long period of time. Problems that reached across government and institutions expanded. Multiple proposals were put on the policy agenda and refined through special commissions and blue-ribbon panels. The reallocation of federal funds for care and access to tax-exempt financing for nonprofit hospitals created "windows of opportunity" and dramatically altered the interests of the city's partnered medical institutions. Focusing events included the *Philadelphia Daily News* exposé of the condition of PGH; the reelection of Mayor Rizzo, who, in his second term, could politically afford to be less concerned with reelection; and the creation of the Hospital Authority of Philadelphia.

PGH: Reconciling the Myth and the Reality

One of the great difficulties in coming to terms with the PGH closure is that, at the time of the closure, the myth of PGH, the public hospital of storied memory, was what remained of a once-noble institution. The reality of PGH—inadequate financing, poor staffing, lack of modernized equipment, intolerable physical plant issues, supply shortages, and intractable bureaucratic complexities that directly impacted patient care—was vastly different from the myth, which was embodied in the hearts and minds of those loyal to PGH. The reality was accurately described, in the most graphic of terms, as a failing institution, whose best days were a part of Philadelphia's history, and could not be part of Philadelphia's future. Those who opposed the closure were loyal to an idea, a concept, that eluded expression, in practical terms, in the day-to-day life of the institution, as the health care world became more of an industry, and the politics of the new benevolence could not sustain the ideal.

The closure of PGH, at the time that it occurred, was a necessary and correct decision. The Alpha Center study findings, applied retrospectively, support this conclusion. But the rationality of facing the health care world as it emerged was, and still is, cold comfort for those who considered PGH more than a hospital. For them, the closure was a capitulation to forces larger than themselves and their principles. For those believers in the mythical PGH, there was, and perhaps still is, no rational argument that could adequately sustain and defend the closure decision.

Lessons Learned and Not Learned

The debate to close PGH often included dialogue and concern for the poor and underserved. At that time, the resolution to close revolved around assumptions that the new entitlement programs—Medicare for the aged and Medicaid for the poor—would cover the bulk of the patient population that used PGH. Moreover, development of a new ambulatory care system and contractual agreements for special services would be able to provide more efficient care in more appropriate settings. And finally, that those needing nursing home beds and skilled care could receive that care, and the fiscal burden on the city would be lessened.

When we "fast-forward" to today, we find that the intractability of some of the problems remain, but are configured differently, with new threats to the integrity of the delivery system and unanticipated consequences of the previous public policy decisions. Since the closure of PGH, the percentage of the Gross National Product spent on health care has increased dramatically, from about 8 percent in 1977 to roughly 14 percent in 2001.[21] Scientific advancements in curing disease, and improving longevity and quality of life, continue apace. But the utopian ideals of benevolent and comprehensive care still elude us. A constant struggle exists between insurers and providers. Managed care plans demand better "management" of patients and their care. Providers insist that the costs of treating patients continue to outstrip their fiscal capacity in the face of a less-than-optimal patient mix, a mix that includes large numbers of managed care/Medicaid and uninsured patients. Providers also face the challenge of dramatically increasing medical malpractice insurance rates that can drive up premiums and marginalize the capacities of physicians and hospitals to manage costs. More middle-class families are losing health care benefits through loss of employment, or copayments or COBRA payments that cannot be met with minimum wage

jobs or unemployment compensation. In Philadelphia neighborhoods, and in towns and neighborhoods across the country where
hospitals provide care to the less affluent, a poor patient population
mix can spell fiscal ruin for many institutions.[22] Hospitals continuing to close are an ongoing reminder: We have yet to solve the problem of how to adequately provide care—safely, benevolently, and
responsibly—for the poor and for those who may be without work to
sustain themselves and their families. Who—or what—will assume
the role of the 21st century almshouse?[23]

The New Jerusalem

If one stands on the corner of Civic Center Boulevard and Osler Cir-
cle and gazes across the landscape of the former PGH site, one cannot help but be struck by the sheer magnitude of size and the critical
mass of scientific discovery, advancement, and health care delivery
and education that still occurs there. Currently located on Osler Cir-
cle are the buildings of the Children's Hospital of Philadelphia, which
include the Leonard and Madelyn Abramson Pediatric Cancer
Research Center; The Children's Hospital of Philadelphia; The Children's Seashore House; and the University of Pennsylvania School of
Nursing. Directly bordering the PGH site are multiple life science
buildings of the University of Pennsylvania, including two new
almost-skyscraper-like biomedical research buildings: Biomedical
Research Buildings II/III, or the BRB towers; the Silverstein Pavilion
for inpatient care; the PENN Towers, providing outpatient services;
the Veterans Affairs Hospital; the Philadelphia Medical Examiner's
Office; and the Consortium, a mental health collaborative. These
institutions are the modern-day temples of medical advancement,
towering in appearance and in intent. Across Civic Center Boulevard,
on the grounds of an earlier incarnation of PGH, a massive plan for
new scientific research and treatment is underway. Children's Hospital of Philadelphia, in concert with the University of Pennsylvania, is
engaged in planning the development of state-of-the-art research and
treatment facilities.

While the physical manifestation of PGH has passed into storied memory, the traditions of achievement, advancement, and scientific excellence remain. What also remains is embodied in the
complexities of financing health care delivery. Enduring are the ever-

asked questions, raised by those who first conceived of the American almshouse: How do we care for, and pay for, the sick, the infirm, the aged, and the less fortunate? Each generation will have to answer these questions for itself. History will judge if we have lived up to the challenges posed by political, social, and scientific philosophers, like John Stuart Mill and Sir William Osler.

For Mill, do we act in concert with the premise that it is our political and social obligation "to perform certain acts of individual beneficence, such as saving a fellow creature's life, or interposing to protect the defenseless against ill-usage. . . A person may cause evil to others not only by his action, but by his inaction, and in either case is justly accountable to them for the injury"?[24] For Osler, do we pursue with intellectual curiosity and vigor, "to wrest from nature the secrets which have perplexed philosophers in all ages to track to their sources the causes of disease"?[25] Just as the founders of the Philadelphia General Hospital grappled with these aspects of the human condition, we, their descendents in science and benevolence, also enjoin the struggle.

Notes

1. See Hoag Levins, "PGH: Death by Neglect...Supply, Staff Shortages Killing Patients," *Philadelphia Daily News*, January 26, 1976; Hoag Levins, "PGH: Shortage of Nurses Endanger Patients," *Philadelphia Daily News*, January 27, 1976; Hoag Levins, "Is PGH Doomed?" *Philadelphia Daily News*, January 30, 1976; letter to Dr. Lewis Bluemle and Dr. Truman Schnabel from David Maxey, Esq., January 5, 1968. UPC 56.5, Box 1, University of Pennsylvania, PGH Archives; see other letters from Maxey to the university dated January 17, February 17, and May 16, 1968. UPC 56.5, Box 1, University of Pennsylvania, PGH Archives.

2. Reports include: Edward V. Sparer, *Medical School Accountability in the Public Hospital: The University of Pennsylvania and the Philadelphia General Hospital* (Unpublished report: Health Law Project, University of Pennsylvania, 1974); Mayor's Committee on Municipal Health Services, *Report of the Mayor's Committee on Municipal Health Services* (Philadelphia: Mayor's Committee on Municipal Health Services, February 1970); JRB Associates, *Impact of the Closing of Philadelphia General Hospital* (McLean, VA, 1979); Joint Committee of Board of Health and Board of Trustees, *Report of the Joint Committee of the Board of Health and PGH Board of Trustees to Consider the Responsibilities of the City of Philadelphia for Personal Health Services, including Care of the Chronically Ill and Aged, and the Role of the Philadelphia General Hospital with Respect to These Responsibilities* (Philadelphia, 1967); City of Philadelphia, *A Comprehensive Report on the Disposition of the Services of Philadelphia General Hospital, as well as the Establishment of the Philadelphia Nursing Home and New and Expanded Programs of the Philadelphia Department of Public Health* (Philadelphia, May 1978); Hospital Survey Committee, *Report and Recommendations of the Hospital Survey Committee with*

Respect to Alternatives for the Provision of Medical Care now Rendered to the Citizens of Philadelphia at Philadelphia General Hospital (Philadelphia, May 1972); Philadelphia Department of Public Health, *Comments and Analysis of Hospital Survey Committee Report on Philadelphia General Hospital of May 2, 1972* (Philadelphia, May 1972); and Medicon Study, *Philadelphia General Hospital Final Report Preliminary Planning, Program of Requirements and Cost Estimates* (Philadelphia, 1976).

3. Medicon Study, executive summary.

4. John O'Donnell, *Commissioned to Serve: A History of the Hospitals and Higher Education Authority of Philadelphia* (Philadelphia: The Vantage Center, 2000), entire book, but especially chapters II and III. Chapter II describes the founding of the authority, and chapter III details the high rate of application to the authority for local nonprofits, described as the opening of "a floodgate" (p. 46). By the end of the first year, 12 local institutions had applied or indicated that they would soon apply for funds that would total over a quarter of a billion dollars.

5. "PGH: Shortage of Nurses Endanger Patients," *Philadelphia Daily News*, January 27, 1976.

6. David Cleary, "PGH 'Inflates' Patient Lists, Polk Admits," *Philadelphia Bulletin*, March 18, 1976. Also see oral interview by author with Eileen Kelly, Philadelphia, July 29, 2003.

7. See oral history interview by author with Stephanie Stachniewicz, Philadelphia, January 25, 2001, and February 15, 2001. Also see Pennsylvania Economy League, *Philadelphia Government*, 6th ed. (Philadelphia, 1963), 128-130.

8. See letters from Maxey to the university dated January 17, February 17, and May 16, 1968. UPC 56.5, Box 1, University of Pennsylvania, PGH Archives.

9. Mayor's Committee on Municipal Hospital Services, *Report of the Mayor's Committee on Municipal Health Services* (Philadelphia, February 1970), 143.

10. "Tate Contacts University Regarding PGH," *The Daily Pennsylvanian*, March 21, 1969.

11. See multiple news reports, noted earlier, by Hoag Levins in the *Philadelphia Daily News*; see the interviews with Stephanie Stachniewicz and Eileen Kelly, which describe their sense of the disconnect between the public view and their lived experiences as nurses at PGH; correspondence and memos from PGH indicate the need to develop a positive public relations campaign to combat the negative profile generated by the bad publicity.

12. S.A. Paolantonio, *Frank Rizzo: The Last Big Man in Big City America* (Philadelphia: Camino Books, 1993), 197-200. Also see Maria K. Mitchell, "Privatizing New York City's Public Hospitals: The Politics of Policy Making" (Ph.D. dissertation, The City University of New York, 1998), which describes the fiscal collapse that necessitated the change in structure. Also see oral history interview by author with Ernest Zeger (Philadelphia, June 22, 2003), the executive director of PGH at the time of the closure, who noted that the New York City bankruptcy was a significant factor in the closure discussion.

13. See oral history interview by author with Walter Lear, Carlisle, PA, June 22, 2003; also see "Court Backs Right to Close PGH," *Philadelphia Bulletin*, August 12, 1976, 1, 6.

14. See the oral history interviews by author with Lenora Berson (Philadelphia, January 5, 2001) and Walter Lear (Philadelphia, July 30, 2003). For background on the political significance of 1199C, see Paolantonio, 193-195.

15. Mayor's Committee on Municipal Hospital Services, 18.

16. MDC Systems Corporation, *A Study of The Philadelphia General Hospital and Philadelphia Health Care Needs and Delivery Systems, Final Report. Prepared for the City of Philadelphia Department of Public Health* (Philadelphia, 1971), iv-8.

17. See oral history interviews with Stephanie Stachniewicz and Eileen Kelly. Kelly discusses the use of the term "dispo," meaning disposition case, as the dominant profile of the PGH patient in her last years as a PGH nursing student.

18. For background on bureaucratic culture, see Ralph Hummel, *The Bureaucratic Experience* (New York: St. Martin's Press, 1987), chapters 2 and 3.

19. Ibid., 137.

20. John W. Kingdon, *Agendas, Alternatives, and Public Policies*, 2nd ed. (New York: Longman, 2003). See entire book, but especially the introduction by James Thurber, and 42-44, 67-70, 113-115, 143-144, 162-164, 194-195.

21. Organization for Economic Cooperation and Development., *OECD Health Data 2003.* Downloaded March 25, 2004, from http://www.oecd.org/dataoecd/10/20/2789777.pdf?channelId=34487&homeChannelId=33717&fileTitle=Health+Data+03%2C+tables+and+charts

22. At the time of this writing, the announcement of the closure of the Medical College of Pennsylvania Hospital in Philadelphia has been made, and is underway, due in substantial part to inadequate reimbursements and case mix of the patient population.

23. It is worth noting that the Philadelphia General Hospital still technically exists. The city's nursing home, which is now run on a contract basis with Episcopal Hospital, is on the city's books as "The Philadelphia General Hospital Nursing Home." This fact could have presented an interesting option for the Rizzo administration, since they could have made a public relations argument that they were returning to the original intention of the almshouse by caring for those most in need with nowhere else to go.

24. John Stuart Mill, "On Liberty," in *The World's Great Thinkers: Man and State, The Political Philosophers*, eds. S. Commins and R. Linscott (New York: Random House, 1947), 146.

25. This quote by Sir William Osler is chiseled into the granite wall of the Abramson Research Building, part of the Children's Hospital of Philadelphia research complex, which now stands on the approximate site of Osler's work in Philadelphia.

Appendix A

TABLE 1

Number of Surviving Hospitals Classified by Type of Ownership and Year of Founding—1946

Year of Founding	Total Hospitals in State	Govt.-Owned (local and state)	Nonprofit Association	Church	Proprietary
1700-1799	2	1	1		
1800-1850	6		4	2	
1851-1860	7	2	2	2	1
1861-1870	9		9		
1871-1880	19	4	12	3	
1881-1890	25	3	18	4	
1891-1900	56	9	44	3	
1901-1910	60	8	41	5	6
1911-1920	51	8	33	3	7
1921-1930	40	8	21	6	14
1931-1940	23	3	10	1	9
1941-1947	24	2	8	2	12
Date Unknown	25	1	6	7	11
Totals	356	49	209	38	60

Adapted from Survey Staff of the Pennsylvania Committee on Hospital Facilities, Organization and Standards, *The Pennsylvania Hospital Survey and Plan* (Harrisburg, 1949).

Appendix B

TABLE 1

Public, Voluntary, and Proprietary Hospitals—1935

	Public Hospitals	Voluntary Hospitals	Proprietary Hospitals	All Hospitals
Average numbers of beds	156	92	23	70
Distribution by number of beds (%)				
Under 25	16.5	11.9	56.7	27.6
25-49	27.6	21.9	26.7	24.2
50-149	29.0	44.9	15.6	33.1
150 and over	26.9	21.3	1.0	15.1
Total	100.0	100.0	100.0	100.0
Community size (%)				
Under 40,000	12.5	39.0	48.5	100.0
40,000-99,999	12.4	57.5	30.1	100.0
100,000-249,000	15.4	61.6	23.0	100.0
250,000 and over	10.9	69.1	20.0	100.0
Source of operating revenue (%)				
Patients	16.7	70.9	91.4	62.4
Taxes	81.0		4.1	23.8
Endowments	0.5	6.3	0.5	0.0
Gifts	1.8	12.5	4.0	13.8
Total	100.0	100.0	100.0	100.0
Equality of access for social classes and income groups	most accessible	intermediate	least accessible	
Rate of occupancy (%)	79	63	45	57
Length of stay (days)	18.3	11.9	9.2	13.1
Assets per bed ($)	3,887	5,483	2,486	4,432
Endowment per bed ($)	144	1,633	127	1,090
Expenses ($)				
Per bed yearly	850	1,198	915	1,073
Per patient day	3.05	5.24	4.44	n.a.
Per patient admission	55.96	65.66	54.83	n.a.
Income per bed, annual ($)	850	1,158	960	1,054
Indicators of quality				
Nurses per bed	0.23	0.38	0.26	0.33
Employees per bed	0.63	0.87	0.56	0.77
Employees per 1,000 patients	800	1,400	1,000	n.a.
Accredited by American College of Surgeons (%)	42.9	57.1	14.8	41.1
Value of equipment per bed ($)	62.60	76.80	45.00	64.18

n.a.=not available

Adapted from J. Hollingsworth and E. Hollingsworth, *Controversy about American Hospitals: Funding, Ownership and Performance* (Washington, DC: American Enterprise Institute for Public Policy Research, 1987), p. 90.

TABLE 2
Public, Voluntary, and Proprietary Hospitals—1961

	Public Hospitals	Voluntary Hospitals	Proprietary Hospitals	All Hospitals
Average number of beds (N=5,021)	124	139	45	121
Distribution by number of beds (%)				
Under 25	10.0	6.7	32.0	11.4
25-49	33.9	20.0	39.6	26.4
50-99	27.4	25.6	19.5	25.1
100-299	20.9	36.1	8.7	28.2
300 or more	7.8	11.6	0.2	8.9
Total	100.0	100.0	100.0	100.0
Source of revenue (%)				
Consumer	58.0	87.1	97.9	81.6
Government	42.0	6.5	2.1	13.7
Philanthropy	—	6.4	—	4.7
Total	100.0	100.0	100.0	100.0
Equality of access for social classes and income groups				
Discharges not paid				
by insurance (%)	43.9	26.9	29.8	32.0
Rate of occupancy (%)	72	76	65	74
Length of stay (days)	8.8	7.5	5.8	7.6
Assets per bed ($) (N=4,186)	11,742	13,440	5,571	12,181
Expenses ($)				
Per bed yearly (N=4,521)	5,811.00	7,161.00	6,232.00	6,715.00
Per patient day	33.29	36.04	32.27	34.98
Per admission	281.69	270.06	194.09	267.38
Revenue per bed ($) (N=4,434)	5,608.00	7,342.00	6,671.00	6,846.00
Indicators of quality				
Full-time-equivalent				
employees per bed	1.6	1.8	1.3	1.7
Residency program approved				
by American Medical				
Association (%) (N=5,042)	11.9	21.6	1.2	16.3
Accreditation, JCAH (%)				
(N=5,042)	44.6	72.1	21.6	58.1
Technological complexity:				
facilities and services average				
(maximum=21) (N=3,973)	10.4	11.9	8.9	11.1

Adapted from J. Hollingsworth and E. Hollingsworth, *Controversy about American Hospitals: Funding, Ownership and Performance* (Washington, DC: American Enterprise Institute for Public Policy Research, 1987), p. 98.

T A B L E   3
Public, Voluntary, and Proprietary Hospitals—1979

	Public Hospitals	Voluntary Hospitals	Proprietary Hospitals	All Hospitals
Average number of beds	116	210	115	169
Distribution by number of beds (%)				
Under 25	7.9	2.9	6.9	4.9
25-49	29.3	12.2	19.3	18.4
50-99	31.8	20.5	26.1	24.7
100-299	22.9	40.7	42.2	35.5
300 or more	8.1	23.7	5.5	16.5
Total	100.0	100.0	100.0	100.0
Source of revenue (%)				
Medicare	34	34	33	33.7
Medicaid	11	7	7	7.5
Blue Cross	n.a.	n.a.	n.a.	16.3
Other insurance	n.a.	n.a.	n.a.	15.6
Other sources	n.a.	n.a.	n.a.	26.9
Total				100.0
Equality of access for social classes and income groups				
(ratio of uncompensated charges to total charges)				
Teaching hospitals	2.77	0.90		
Nonteaching hospitals	1.41	0.79	0.65	
Rate of occupancy (%)	69.1	76.5	63.9	73.8
Length of stay (days) (N=5,750)	7.7	8.0	6.6	7.7
Assets per bed ($)	43,437.00	48,883.00	40,375.00	47,010.00
Expenses ($)				
Per bed yearly	62,573.00	69,492.00	57,840.00	67,009.00
Per patient day	205.10	217.93	225.87	215.75
Per patient admission	1,524.24	1,681.70	1,477.33	1,632.16
Revenue per inpatient day ($)	n.a.	253.67	n.a.	249.84
Indicators of quality (N=5,750)				
Full-time-equivalent				
employees per bed	2.7	2.9	2.1	2.8
Residency program approved				
by American Medical				
Association (%)	9.5	21.5	1.2	15.2

Adapted from J. Hollingsworth & E. Hollingsworth, *Controversy about American Hospitals: Funding, Ownership and Performance* (Washington, DC: American Enterprise Institute for Public Policy Research, 1987), p. 104.

Appendix C

Manuscript Collections

City of Philadelphia Archive

Files of past officials and departments of the City of Philadelphia
  • Correspondence and memoranda arranged by subject and date
Minutes of official executive meetings
PGH Board of Trustees minutes
Reports or surveys that were published for external distribution
City-wide records schedule

Center for the Study of Nursing History
University of Pennsylvania
Philadelphia, Pennsylvania

Personal collection of Stephanie Stachniewicz, former director of nursing
    at PGH
Financing of Hospital Care in the United States, Volumes I-III

College of Physicians
Philadelphia, Pennsylvania

PGH medical library, including photographs depicting its history
Osler Memorial Committee collection
Alice Fisher's Duty Register of the training school for nursing
Philadelphia Hospital Reports

Hospitals Authority of Philadelphia
Philadelphia, Pennsylvania

Material related to hospital financing in the City of Philadelphia

Institute of Social Medicine and Community Health
Philadelphia, Pennsylvania

Repository of Dr. Walter Lear's personal collection
Fellowship Commission report

Dr. Lewis Polk
Doylestown, Pennsylvania

Reports
- Board of Health
- Board of Trustees
- The Mayor's Committee on Municipal Health Services
- Hospital Survey Committee
- MDC Systems reports of the Division of Health and Human Services
- Medicon, Inc.

City press releases

Newspaper and journal articles from period preceding and following closure

Correspondence and progress reports from the Managing Director to City Council

University of Pennsylvania
Philadelphia, Pennsylvania

24 boxes of files devoted to PGH
- Correspondence between the medical school and PGH/City of Philadelphia and correspondence between legal counsel and the University regarding PGH contracts
- Internal University administrative records, memoranda, minutes from multiple internal committee meetings
- PGH Board of Trustees minutes

Urban Archive Center
Temple University
Philadelphia, Pennsylvania

Oral History Project—key informant interviews with individuals influential in PGH and/or the closure

Philadelphia Bulletin Morgue

Appendix D

Interviews

Lenora Berson, active member of Americans for Democratic Action, January 5, 2001, Philadelphia, Pennsylvania

Lt. Anthony Fulwood, police officer and former member of Rizzo's security unit, July 23, 2003, Philadelphia, Pennsylvania

Eileen (Duffy) Kelly, student president of the last graduating class of the School of Nursing of PGH, July 29, 2003, Philadelphia, Pennsylvania

Judge Isador Kranzel, former Deputy City Solicitor, February 17, 2004, Philadelphia, Pennsylvania

Dr. Walter Lear, former Deputy Health Commissioner, July 30, 2003, Philadelphia, Pennsylvania

Hillel Levinson, former Managing Director of the City of Philadelphia during the Rizzo administration, February 19, 2004, Philadelphia, Pennsylvania

Dr. Lewis Polk, acting Health Commissioner during Rizzo administration, December 11, 2000, Philadelphia, Pennsylvania

Commissioner Joseph Rizzo, former Fire Commissioner during the Rizzo administration, June 25, 2003, Philadelphia, Pennsylvania

Barry Savitz, former health center manager in the Department of Public Health during the Rizzo administration, July 26, 2000, Philadelphia, Pennsylvania

Stephanie Stachniewicz, former Director of Nursing for PGH and PGH School of Nursing, January 25 and February 15, 2001, Philadelphia, Pennsylvania

Duncan Van Dusen, former Assistant Dean of the University of Pennsylvania Medical School, June 18, 2003, Philadelphia, Pennsylvania

Martin Weinberg, former City Solicitor and political advisor to Mayor Rizzo, July 28, 2003, Philadelphia, Pennsylvania

Tina Weintraub, former Executive Director of PGH, August 7, 2000, Philadelphia, Pennsylvania

Ernest Zeger, former Administrative Services Director and acting Executive Director of PGH, June 22, 2003, Carlisle, Pennsylvania

At the completion of this project, transcripts and tapes will be stored at the Center for Nursing History at the University of Pennsylvania.

Bibliography

Baker, P. "The Domestication of Politics: Women and American Political Society, 1780-1920," in *Women, the State, and Welfare*, ed. L. Gordon (Madison: University of Wisconsin Press, 1990).

"Belt-Tightening at Charity," *The Times Picayune*, July 28, 2002.

Beschloss, Michael. *Taking Charge: Johnson White House Tapes, 1963-1964* (New York: Simon & Schuster, 1997).

Blaisdell, F.W. "Development of the City-County (Public) Hospital," *Archives of Surgery* 129 (1994): 760-764.

Bovbjerg, Randall R., Jill A. Marsteller, and Frank C. Ullman. *Health Care for the Poor and Uninsured after a Public Hospital's Closure or Conversion* (Washington, D.C.: The Urban Institute, 2000).

Bugbee, George. *Recollections of a Good Life: An Autobiography* (Chicago: American Hospital Association, The Hospital Research and Educational Trust, 1987).

Camper, Anne B., Larry S. Gage, Barbara Eyman, and Steven K. Stranne. *The Safety Net in Transition, Monograph II: Reforming the Legal Structure and Governance of Safety Net Hospitals* (Washington, DC: National Association of Public Hospitals and Health Systems, 1996).

City of Philadelphia. *A Comprehensive Report on the Disposition of the Services of Philadelphia General Hospital, as well as the Establishment of the Philadelphia Nursing Home and New and Expanded Programs of the Philadelphia Department of Public Health* (Philadelphia, 1978).

Clayton, Lillian. "School of Nursing," in *The History of Blockley*, ed. John Welsh Croskey (Philadelphia: F.A. Davis, 1929).

Cleary, David M. "Decision on PGH Final, Mayor Says," *Philadelphia Bulletin*, February 18, 1976.

_____. "Ethel Allen Outlines Steps to Save PGH," *Philadelphia Bulletin*, February 22, 1976.

_____. "PGH Plans are 'Fluid,' Health Council Told," *Philadelphia Bulletin*, February 26, 1976.

Commission on Public-General Hospitals. *The Future of the Public-General Hospital: An Agenda for Transition* (Chicago: Hospital Research and Educational Trust, 1978).

"Court Backs Right to Close PGH." *Philadelphia Bulletin*, August 12, 1976.

Croskey, John Welsh. *History of Blockley* (Philadelphia: F.A. Davis, 1929).

Da Costa, J. Chalmers. "The Old Blockley Hospital: Its Characters and Characteristics," in *The History of Blockley*, ed. John Welsh Croskey (Philadelphia: F.A. Davis, 1929).

The Daily Pennsylvanian, "Judge Overturns Ban on Rizzo's Decision to Close PGH," February 25, 1976.

Dallek, Robert. *Flawed Giant: Lyndon B. Johnson, 1960-1973* (New York: Oxford University Press, 1998).

_____. *An Unfinished Life: John F. Kennedy, 1917-1963* (Boston: Little Brown, 2003).

David, Gunter. "3 Councilmen Urge Big Meeting on PGH," The Philadelphia Bulletin, February 27, 1976.

_____. "Protesters Join Forces to Blitz City Hall," *Philadelphia Bulletin*, March 12, 1976.

David, Gunter and John Dubois. "Meetings, Hearings Planned on PGH," *Philadelphia Bulletin*, February 20, 1976.

Dieckmann, Janet. *Caring for the Chronically Ill: Philadelphia, 1945-1965*, ed. Stuart Bruchey (New York: Garland Publishing, 1999).

Drake, D. "Hospital Saga: Years of Neglect Breed Shortages, Low Morale," *Philadelphia Inquirer*, December 8, 1970.

Dowling, H.F. *City Hospitals: The Undercare of the Underprivileged* (Cambridge, MA: Harvard University Press, 1982).

Drake, Donald. "While Awaiting a Plan for PGH, Some Speculation," *Philadelphia Inquirer*, March 21, 1976.

Fairman, Julie and Joan Lynaugh. *Critical Care Nursing: A History* (Philadelphia: University of Pennsylvania Press, 1998).

Financing of Hospital Care in the United States, Volume I: Factors Affecting the Cost of Hospital Care, ed. John Hayes (New York: Blakiston, 1954).

Financing of Hospital Care in the United States, Volume II: Prepayment and the Community, ed. John Hayes (New York: Blakiston, 1954).

Financing of Hospital Care in the United States, Volume III: Financing Hospital Care for Non-Wage and Low-Income Groups, ed. John Hayes (New York: Blakiston, 1954).

Gibson, Mary Barnett. "What's Past Is Prologue," in *The Columbia World of Quotations* (New York: Columbia University Press, 1996).

Gillespie, John T. "Union Leaders Organize March to Protest PGH Closing Plan," *Philadelphia Bulletin*, February 18, 1976.

Grele, Robert J. *Envelopes of Sound: The Art of Oral History*, 2nd ed. (New York: Praeger, 1991).

Harrington, Michael. *The Other America* (New York: Scribner, 1997).

Himmelfarb, Gertrude. *On Liberty and Liberalism: The Case Study of John Stuart Mill* (New York: Random House Children's Books, 1974).

Hollingsworth, J. and E. Hollingsworth. *Controversy about American Hospitals: Funding, Ownership and Performance* (Washington D.C.: American Enterprise Institute for Public Policy Research, 1987).

Hospital Survey Committee. *Report and Recommendations of the Hospital Survey Committee with Respect to Alternatives for the Provision of Medical Care Now Rendered to the Citizens of Philadelphia at Philadelphia General Hospital* (Philadelphia, 1972).

Howell, Martha and Walter Prevenier. *From Reliable Sources: An Introduction to Historical Methods* (Ithaca, NY: Cornell University Press, 2001).

Hummel, Ralph. *The Bureaucratic Experience* (New York: St. Martin's Press, 1987).

Isaacs, M., K. Lichter, and C. Lipschultz. *The Urban Public Hospital: Options for the 1980's* (Bethesda, MD: Alpha Center, 1982).

Irving, Washington. "Westminister Abbey," in *American Quotations*, eds. Gorton Carruth and Eugene Ehrlich (Avenel, NJ: Wing Books, 1992).

Jefferson, Thomas, in *American Quotations*, eds. Gorton Carruth and Eugene Ehrlich (Avenel, NJ: Wing Books, 1992).

Joint Committee of Board of Health and Board of Trustees. *Report of the Joint Committee of the Board of Health and PGH Board of Trustees to Consider the Responsibilities of the City of Philadelphia for Personal Health Services, including Care of the Chronically Ill and Aged, and the Role of the Philadelphia General Hospital with Respect to These Responsibilities* (Philadelphia, 1967).

JRB Associates. *Impact of the Closing of Philadelphia General Hospital* (McLean, VA, 1979).

Jones, Diana Nelson. "Appalachia's War: The Poorest of the Poor Struggle Back," *Pittsburgh Post Gazette*, November 26, 2000.

Katz, Michael B. *In the Shadow of the Poorhouse: A Social History of Welfare in America* (New York: Basic Books, 1986).

_____. *The Undeserving Poor: From the War on Poverty to the War on Welfare* (New York: Pantheon Books, 1989).

Kingdon, John. *Agendas, Alternatives, and Public Policies*, 2nd ed. (New York: Longman, 2003).

Levins, Hoag. "City Slowly Strangling Hospital, Says Staff," *Philadelphia Daily News*, January 30, 1976.

_____. "Historic Hospital Hardly a Bicen Shrine," *Philadelphia Daily News*, January 27, 1976.

_____. "Inside PGH," *Philadelphia Daily News*, January 28, 1976.

_____. "Is PGH Doomed?" *The Philadelphia Daily News*, January 30, 1976.

_____. "Legislator Asks for PGH Probe," *Philadelphia Bulletin*, February 21, 1976.

_____. "PGH Chairman Sells to His Own Hospital," *Philadelphia Daily News*, January 28, 1976.

_____. "PGH: Death by Neglect. . . Supply, Staff Shortages Killing Patients," *Philadelphia Daily News*, January 26, 1976.

_____. "PGH Flunks PA Standard, Still Licensed," *Philadelphia Daily News*, January 28, 1976.

_____. "PGH: Shortage of Nurses Endanger Patients," *Philadelphia Daily News*, January 27, 1976.

_____. "Prosecution at PGH?" *Philadelphia Daily News*, January 31, 1976.

_____. "Nurse-Juggling Act Hid Shortage from HEW," *Philadelphia Daily News*, January 27, 1976.

_____. "State Knew PGH Was Coming Up Short," *Philadelphia Daily News*, February 10, 1976.

_____. "Survey After Survey, and Yet No Action," *Philadelphia Daily News*, January 29, 1976.

_____. "Watchdog Agency to Inspect PGH," *Philadelphia Daily News*, February 11, 1976.

Long, Huey P. *Every Man a King* (Chicago: Quadrangle Books, 1964).

Ludmerer, K.M. *Time to Heal: American Medical Education from the Turn of the Century to the Era of Managed Care* (New York: Oxford University Press, 1999).

Lynaugh, Joan E. "From Respectable Domesticity to Medical Efficiency: The Changing Kansas City Hospital, 1875-1920," in *The American General Hospital: Communities and Social Contexts*, eds. D.E. Long and J. Golden (Ithaca, NY: Cornell University Press, 1989).

Mayor's Committee on Municipal Health Services. *Report of the Mayor's Committee on Municipal Health Services* (Philadelphia, 1970).

McBride, David. *Integrating the City of Medicine: Blacks in Philadelphia Health Care, 1910-1965* (Philadelphia: Temple University Press, 1989).

McCullough, David G. *Truman* (New York: Simon & Schuster, 1993).

McPherson, James. "The Second American Revolution," in *Major Problems in the Civil War and Reconstruction*, ed. Michael Perman (Boston: Houghton Mifflin, 1998).

MDC Systems Corporation. *A Study of the Philadelphia General Hospital and Philadelphia Health Care Needs and Delivery Systems, Final Report. Prepared for the City of Philadelphia Department of Public Health* (Philadelphia, 1971).

Medicon. *Philadelphia General Hospital Final Report: Preliminary Planning, Program of Requirements and Cost Estimates* (Philadelphia, 1976).

Mill, John Stuart. "On Liberty," in *The World's Greatest Thinkers: Man and State, Political Philosophers*, eds. Saxe Commins & Robert N. Linscott (New York: Random House, 1947).

_____. *On Liberty*, ed. Gertrude Himmelfarb (New York: Penguin Classics, 1976).

Mills, Charles K. "The Philadelphia Almshouse and Philadelphia Hospital from 1854 to 1908," in *The History of Blockley*, ed. John Welsh Croskey (Philadelphia: F.A. Davis, 1929).

Mitchell, Maria K. "Privatizing New York City's Public Hospitals: The Politics of Policy Making" (Ph.D. dissertation, The City University of New York, 1998).

National Forum on Hospital and Health Affairs. *The Changing Composition of the Hospital System* (Durham, NC: Duke University Press, 1969).

O'Donnell, John. *Commissioned to Serve: A History of the Hospitals and Higher Education Authority* (Philadelphia: The Vantage Center, 2000).

Organization for Economic Cooperation and Development. OECD Health Data 2003. http://www.oecd.org/dataoecd/10/20/2789777.pdf?channelld= 34487&homeChannelld=33717&fileTitle=Health+Data_03%2C+tables+ and+charts

Paolantonio, S.A. *Frank Rizzo: The Last Big Man in Big City America* (Philadelphia: Camino Books, 1993).

The Pennsylvania Economy League. *Philadelphia Government*, 6th ed. (Philadelphia, 1963).

Philadelphia Bulletin, "5 on Council Hit Lack of Data on PGH," April 20, 1976.

_____, "19 Hospitals to Aid Patients," April 30, 1977.

_____, "Chaplain Won't Give Up Until the Doors Are Shut," October 10, 1976.

_____, "City Striving to Reach Pact on PGH Patients," April 29, 1976.

_____, "Court OKs End of PGH," August 13, 1976.

_____, "Future for PGH Male Nurse: City Offers Him Janitor Job," May 29, 1977.

_____, "Hearse Leads March to Protest PGH Closing," May 23, 1976.

_____, "Hospitals Ask for More City Aid," May 3, 1976.

_____, "Hospitals Ease Off on PGH," May 2, 1976.

_____, "Issues in PGH March," February 25, 1976.

_____, "Judge Ruling Allows Closing of PGH," February 24, 1976.

_____, "Last Patients Transferred from PGH," June 18, 1977.

_____, "Many PGH Doctors, Nurses are Leaving," May 5, 1976.

_____, "March to Protest Closing of PGH," May 11, 1976.

_____, "Marchers Protest PGH Closing Plan," February 26, 1976.

_____, "Maternity Service at PGH Closed," September 30, 1976.

_____, "Old Blockely Nurses: Pride, Tradition Live On in the Double Frill Cap," May 19, 1977.

_____, "PGH 'Inflates' Patient Lists, Polk Admits," March 18, 1976.

_____, "PGH Outpatient Services to be Moved to Centers," September 1, 1976.

_____, "Phila to Transfer 86 When Laundry Sold," April 30, 1976.

_____, "Protest Crowd Chants Recall," February 25, 1976.

_____, "Rizzo Reaffirms Private Hospitals Will Care for Poor," October 20, 1976.

_____, "Schwartz Seeks Parlay on PGH," February 18, 1976.

_____, "When PGH Closes, Regulars Will Lose," May 2, 1977.

Philadelphia Daily News, "42 Staff Doctors Demand Action at PGH," February 3, 1976.

_____, "City Poor: PGH Crisis Pawns," May 14, 1976.

_____, "PGH Closing Costs," June 14, 1976.

_____, "PGH: The City Pulled the Plug," May 13, 1976.

_____, "PGH Plan is Still Being Planned," July 7, 1976.

_____, "The PGH Shutdown Proceeds," April 14, 1977.

Philadelphia Department of Public Health. *Comments and Analysis of Hospital Survey Committee Report on Philadelphia General Hospital of May 2, 1972* (Philadelphia, 1972).

Philadelphia Hospital Reports, Volume I, eds. Charles Mills and James Walk (Philadelphia: J.B. Lippincott, 1890).

Philadelphia Hospital Reports, Volume II, eds. Roland G. Curtin and Daniel Hughes (Philadelphia: J.B. Lippincott, 1900).

Philadelphia Inquirer, "City Finds Ways to Soften Loss of PGH," March 27, 1977.

_____, "The PGH Battle," March 1, 1976.

_____, "Problems with the PGH Problem," December 14, 1976.

Reverby, Susan. *Ordered to Care: The Dilemma of American Nursing, 1850-1945* (New York: Cambridge University Press, 1987).

Rosenberg, Charles E. *The Care of Strangers: The Rise of America's Hospital System* (Baltimore: The Johns Hopkins University Press, 1987).

_____. "Community and Communities: The Evolution of the American Hospital," in *The American General Hospital: Communities and Social Contexts*, eds. Diana E. Long and Janet Golden (Ithaca, NY: Cornell University Press, 1989).

_____. *Explaining Epidemics and Other Studies in the History of Medicine* (Cambridge, UK: Cambridge University Press, 1992).

_____. "Social Class and Medical Care in 19th-Century America: The Rise and Fall of the Dispensary," in *Sickness and Health in America: Readings in the History of Medicine and Public Health*, eds. Judith Walzer Leavitt and Ronald L. Numbers, 3rd ed. (Madison: University of Wisconsin Press, 1998).

Rosner, D. *A Once Charitable Enterprise: Hospitals and Health Care in Brooklyn and New York, 1885-1915* (Princeton, NJ: Princeton University Press, 1982).

_____. "Doing Well or Doing Good: The Ambivalent Focus of Hospital Administration," in *The American General Hospital: Communities and Social Contexts*, eds. D.E. Long and J. Golden (Ithaca, NY: Cornell University Press, 1989).

Shesol, Jeffrey. *Mutual Contempt: Lyndon Johnson, Robert Kennedy, and the Feud That Defined a Decade* (New York: W.W. Norton, 1997).

Singer, Ingrid, Lindsay Davison, and Lynne Fagnani. *America's Safety Net Hospitals and Health Systems: Results of the 2001 Annual Member Survey* (Washington, DC: National Association of Public Hospitals and Health Systems, 2003).

Skowronek, S. *Building a New American State: The Expansion of National Administrative Capacities, 1877-1920* (New York: Cambridge University Press, 1982).

Sparer, Edward. *Medical School Accountability in the Public General Hospital: The University of Pennsylvania and the Philadelphia General Hospital* (Philadelphia, The Health Law Project, University of Pennsylvania, 1974).

Spencer, Gil. "Editorial," *Philadelphia Daily News*, February 3, 1976.

Stachniewicz, Stephanie A. and J.K. Axelrod. *The Double Frill: The History of the Philadelphia General Hospital and the School of Nursing* (Philadelphia: George F. Stickley, 1978).

Starr, P. *The Social Transformation of American Medicine: The Rise of a Sovereign Profession and the Making of a Vast Industry* (New York: Basic Books, 1982).

Stevens, Rosemary. *American Medicine and the Public Interest* (New Haven, CT: Yale University Press, 1976).

_____. *In Sickness and in Wealth: American Hospitals in the Twentieth Century* (New York: Basic Books, 1989).

Stone, Chuck. "PGH: The Making and Destroying of Niggers," *Philadelphia Daily News*, February 3, 1976.

Survey Staff of the Pennsylvania Committee on Hospital Facilities, Organization and Standards. *The Pennsylvania Hospital Survey and Plan* (Harrisburg, 1949).

Unger, I. and D. Unger. *LBJ: A Life* (New York: John Wiley & Sons, 1999).

Vansina, Jan. *Oral Tradition as History* (Madison: University of Wisconsin Press, 1985).

Vogel, Morris J. "Patrons, Practitioners, and Patients: The Voluntary Hospital in Mid-Victorian Boston," in *Sickness and Health in America: Readings in the History of Medicine and Public Health*, eds. Judith Walzer Leavitt and Ronald L. Numbers, 3rd ed. (Madison: University of Wisconsin Press, 1997).

Weissman, J. "Uncompensated Hospital Care. Will It Be There If We Need It?" *Journal of the American Medical Association* 276 (October 1996): 823-828.

Welles, Elaine. "NAACP Asks to Place PGH Under Receivership," *Philadelphia Tribune*, January 31, 1976.

_____. "NAACP Hits Filthy, Unsafe Conditions at Philadelphia General," *Philadelphia Tribune*, February 7, 1976.

White, J. William. "Alice Fisher," in *Philadelphia Hospital Reports, Volume II*, eds. C.K. Mills and J.W. Walk (Philadelphia: J.B. Lippincott, 1893).

Wofford, Harris. *Of Kennedys and Kings: Making Sense of the Sixties* (New York: Farrar, Straus & Giroux, 1980).

Women, the State and Welfare, ed. Linda Gordon (Madison: University of Wisconsin Press, 1990).

Yow, Valerie Raleigh. *Recording Oral History: A Practical Guide for Social Scientists* (Thousand Oaks, CA: Sage Publications, 1994).